Pioneering Pathways in Long-Term Care Research and Innovation

Edited by Wilson Abreu

Published in London, United Kingdom

Pioneering Pathways in Long-Term Care Research and Innovation
http://dx.doi.org/10.5772/intechopen.1008635
Edited by Wilson Abreu

Contributors
Akpan Margaret Inemiesit, Audra T. Williams, Donnette A. Wright, Efut Joseph Ajah, Elaunire Monica Agianipe, Emmanuel Edet Udontre, Fatma Abdalla Mohamed Abdalla, Gaotswake Patience Kovane, Hiromi Nakamura-Thomas, Keletwaetse Sakwape, Miriam Mmamphamo Moagi, MiriamM Moagi, Natoya Wade, Ndep Antor Odu, Nobuyuki Sano, Undie Emmanuel Ugbong, Wada Gaolaolwe, Wilson Abreu

First published in London, United Kingdom, 2026 by IntechOpen
IntechOpen is the global imprint of INTECHOPEN LIMITED, registered in England and Wales, registration number: 11086078, 167-169 Great Portland Street, London, W1W 5PF, United Kingdom

For EU product safety concerns: IN TECH d.o.o., Prolaz Marije Krucifikse Kozulić 3, 51000 Rijeka, Croatia, info@intechopen.com or visit our website at intechopen.com.

British Library Cataloguing-in-Publication Data
A catalogue record for this book is available from the British Library

Pioneering Pathways in Long-Term Care Research and Innovation
Edited by Wilson Abreu
p. cm.

This title is part of the Public Health Book Series, Volume 12
Series Editor: José Antonio Mirón Canelo

Print ISBN 978-1-83635-887-9
Online ISBN 978-1-83635-886-2
eBook (PDF) ISBN 978-1-83635-888-6
ISSN 3049-8872

If disposing of this product, please recycle the paper responsibly.

IntechOpen Book Series
Public Health
Volume 12

Aims and Scope of the Series

Public health is what we as a society do collectively to contribute to and ensure the health and social conditions for the enjoyment of health as a resource for life. It can also be defined as science and research that promotes health, prevents disease, and improves populations' well-being and quality of life. Its objective is to know the risk factors that determine and condition the populations' health levels at present. At the end of the 20th century and the beginning of the 21st century, it is unjustifiable and regrettable that morbimortality according to age plays a leading role when the causes are mostly well known and therefore preventable, such as obesity, AIDS, cirrhosis, diabetes mellitus, addictions and cancer associated with the consumption of tobacco and alcohol, etc. In short, public health is science based on epidemiology and biostatistics, and currently, new technologies and artificial intelligence must be incorporated to identify patterns and trends in what we do collectively as a society to ensure living conditions and prevent risk factors that affect individual and population health. For all these reasons, it is essential to scientifically investigate and act on the determinants that impede the well-being and quality of life related to the health of people, patients, and populations in general, given that to control the determinants of diseases, it is important to control the environment and genetics. Consequently, the current fight for public health must prioritize the control of the environment, such as atmospheric and biological pollution and environmental and social biodiversity, promoting the sensitivity and training of society and its individuals by empowering them to make free and appropriate decisions about these aspects to lead healthy lifestyles based on motivation and responsibility in the face of the challenges they cope with from an individual point of view, such as dealing with the addictions that exist in today's complex world. Public health also requires an ethical vision and incorporates strategies to reduce social inequality.

Meet the Series Editor

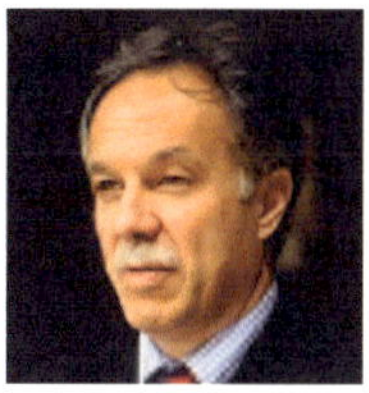

José Antonio Mirón Canelo is a physician, doctor, and professor of Preventive Medicine and Public Health at the Faculty of Medicine and Dentistry of the University of Salamanca with over 30 years of experience. He is the director of the USAL's Expert Degree in Health Management, currently in its 13th edition. Prof. Mirón Canelo directs a research group at the Research Institute of Biomedical Sciences (IBSAL) of the University of Salamanca focused on addressing the challenges and care needs of vulnerable people and patients such as the elderly with multiple pathologies and people with disabilities and dependence. As a teacher, he has been recognized for excellence in teaching three times in a period of five years.

Meet the Volume Editor

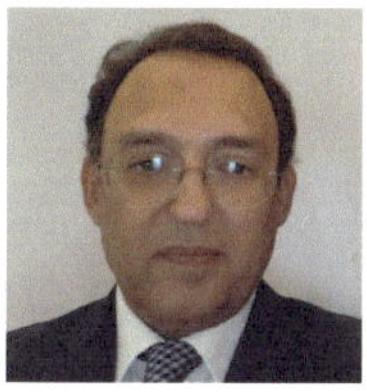

Wilson Correia de Abreu is a Full Professor at the Porto School of Nursing, University of Porto, where he serves as President of the Scientific Council. His academic foundation includes a Ph.D. from the University of Lisbon and the esteemed title of Aggregation, conferred by the University of Aveiro (Health Sciences), which underpins his specialized expertise in Mental Health and Psychiatry. In his academic leadership, Professor Abreu coordinates the Master's program in Mental Health and Psychiatry. His substantive research portfolio is pursued within two key institutional frameworks: the RISE-Health research center at the University of Porto's Faculty of Medicine and the Clinic and Epidemiology of Infectious and Parasitic Diseases (CEDIP) research unit. His investigative focus encompasses several pivotal domains, including mental health epidemiology, HIV/AIDS, palliative and end-of-life care, and the translational application of artificial intelligence and data mining techniques to complex healthcare challenges. This scholarly activity is characterized by an extensive and active international collaboration network that engages peers across all European Union member states, as well as in Norway, Turkey, Brazil, Japan, China, and Australia. Complementing his research and teaching, Professor Abreu has significant experience as an academic administrator and a recognized international consultant, contributing to higher education governance and quality assurance frameworks worldwide. His scholarly output is evidenced by a corpus of influential books and numerous articles in internationally refereed journals, as well as dedicated service on the editorial boards of several prominent academic publications. Linguistically proficient, he is fluent in Portuguese, English, French, and Spanish and maintains basic communicative competence in Italian and Russian, which further facilitates his wide-ranging international academic engagements and discourse.

Contents

Preface

This volume offers a bold and necessary reconceptualization of Long-Term Care (LTC), moving decisively beyond its traditional framing as a monolithic, demographic-driven policy burden. It presents LTC not as a singular challenge but as a complex, lived reality, a dynamic intersection where intimate familial bonds, deep-seated cultural norms, and the structural capacities (or failures) of health systems converge. Through a multifaceted exploration across six distinct yet interconnected chapters, this work synthesizes a cohesive and urgent argument: the global crisis in LTC is, at its core, a crisis of imagination. The prevailing model, fixated on reactive, institutional, and medically-centric responses to physical decline, is fundamentally obsolete. The path forward demands a radical shift towards a proactive, holistic, and culturally embedded care ecosystem. This new paradigm must be engineered to strategically empower informal caregivers as co-producers of health, integrate prevention as its cornerstone, relentlessly pursue deinstitutionalization, and demonstrate profound cultural competence. The following synthesis strategically weaves each chapter's contributions into this overarching thesis, framing a collective discourse that is both academically rigorous and intentionally disruptive.

Central to this reimagined ecosystem is a transformative view of the informal caregiver as a pioneer and structural pillar of the system. Moving far beyond token recognition, this volume posits family members as primary agents of innovation and daily clinical management. Their strategic empowerment, through community-based, culturally tailored education and formal support, is reframed from a complementary welfare consideration to an essential investment in systemic sustainability and quality. This professionalization of the caregiver role is a foundational step, transforming them from an invisible resource into a recognized and skilled protagonist within the care continuum.

This reconceptualization logically demands a second bold expansion: extending the very scope of LTC beyond aging. The book argues compellingly that prolonged dependency and complex care needs are not exclusive to later life. By integrating chronic behavioral health conditions, such as substance use disorders, into the LTC framework, it forces systems to confront and support families navigating highly stigmatized psychosocial crises. This expansion challenges the siloed nature of health and social services, advocating for a system capable of addressing the full spectrum of long-term human vulnerability with integrated mental health and social support.

Underpinning this broader scope is the critical need to address the central paradox of longevity. The celebrated extension of life expectancy, when coupled with a parallel rise in years lived with disability, creates unsustainable pressure on families and systems. This volume positions this paradox not as an inevitable outcome but as the defining systemic challenge of our time. Consequently, it places proactive risk management, targeting modifiable predictors like nutritional status and mobility from mid-life onwards, at the very heart of the LTC agenda. This shifts the system's orientation from costly late-stage intervention to early, sustained prevention, aiming to compress morbidity and alleviate future care burdens.

Operationalizing this vision requires a strategic imperative for deinstitutionalization, recast not merely as an economic necessity but as a core strategy for optimizing the entire health ecosystem. The proposed shift of care delivery from hospitals to domestic and community settings is a deliberate re-engineering of resource flows. It serves the dual strategic objective of liberating acute-care hospital beds for their most efficient use while delivering basic, comfort-focused, and dignity-preserving care in the preferred environment of the individual. This redefines systemic efficiency not through narrow cost-cutting, but through the intelligent allocation of resources to maximize both clinical outcomes for acute conditions and quality of life for chronic ones.

The successful execution of this community-based model depends on cultural competence as a non-negotiable prerequisite. Drawing powerful lessons from global health, the work demonstrates that imposing standardized, top-down models is a recipe for failure. True efficacy and community acceptance are achieved only through the respectful harmonization of evidence-based practices with local traditions and beliefs. This principle elevates community co-creation from a consultative accessory to a fundamental design requirement, rendering obsolete the notion of a one-size-fits-all LTC blueprint.

This volume contends that overcoming the current LTC impasse transcends debates about funding formulas or demographic projections. The primary barrier is a profound crisis of imagination. The book is thus a call to arms, a challenge to policymakers, scholars, and practitioners to abandon incremental adjustments and dare to conceive systems that are simultaneously scientifically robust and deeply relational. It advocates for the construction of resilient, integrated support networks that uphold human dignity across the lifespan, firmly anchored in the strengths of primary care, the comfort of home, and the fabric of community. This is the ambitious, holistic, and necessary reimagining proposed in the pages that follow.

After the Introductory Chapter, the volume continues with Chapter 2: *Perspective Chapter: Family Caregivers - Pioneering Pathways in Long-Term Care Innovation and Research,* which explores the critical role of non-professional family caregivers and assesses their awareness, attitudes, and educational needs in chronic illness care. It concludes that significant gaps in caregiver training undermine their efficacy, positioning the empowerment of caregivers through community-based, culturally tailored educational interventions as a foundational strategy for improving patient outcomes and reducing systemic burdens. This establishes the family unit as the indispensable cornerstone of long-term care systems worldwide.

In Chapter 3: *Global Burden of Lifestyle Diseases and Pressure Injuries: Nutritional Predictors and Impact on Family Health Outcomes*, the authors analyze the public health impact of chronic diseases and pressure injuries among aging populations. It highlights the paradox of longevity, in which longer life spans are associated with greater disability and caregiver strain. It concludes that nutritional status and mobility are critical, modifiable predictors of morbidity. For long-term care, this underscores the need to integrate proactive, prevention-oriented strategies—such as active screening and nutritional support—to mitigate burdens and preserve family well-being.

Turning to a frequently overlooked dimension, Chapter 4: *Crushed by Caregiving: The Growing Burden on Families of Individuals with Substance Use Addiction* delineates the emotional, financial, and social burdens borne by these families. It concludes that caregiving for addiction involves profound role strain exacerbated by stigma and a systemic lack of resources, arguing that a comprehensive long-term care framework must broaden its scope beyond aging to include chronic behavioral health conditions. This expansion necessitates integrated mental health services and anti-stigma initiatives to support vulnerable caregivers.

Chapter 5: *Perspective Chapter: Cultural Patterns and Outcomes of Umbilical Cord Care in Africa - Implications for Neonatal Health and Long-Term Development* critically examines the impact of traditional practices on neonatal outcomes. The investigation finds that while some traditions elevate health risks, the culturally insensitive imposition of biomedical interventions is ineffective. Its key conclusion is that sustainable improvement requires harmonizing evidence-based practices with respected cultural traditions, underscoring a core principle for long-term care: cultural competence and community co-creation are prerequisites for effective care across the life course.

Focusing on a specific socio-cultural context, Chapter 6: *Navigating Caregiving and Work: Key Psychosocial Predictors of Quality of Life amidst Familism in Japan's Evolving Long-Term Care System* aims to identify predictors of quality of life for working caregivers and explore culturally congruent support strategies. It concludes that in contexts of strong familism, burdens disproportionately fall on women, creating conflicts between employment, social participation, and care duties. The chapter argues that systemic resilience depends on culturally attuned interventions, including flexible employment policies, to prevent caregiver burnout and sustain the informal care workforce.

Chapter 7: *Perspective Chapter: Moving Long-Term Care into Home, Community and Primary Healthcare Settings Amid Resource Constraints in Developing Nations* proposes a viable, integrated model for long-term care in resource-constrained settings. It concludes that a decentralized, community-based model integrated with primary healthcare is culturally preferred, dignity-preserving, and cost-effective. This model, which recommends policy redesign for "aging in place" and capacity building for community workers, presents a strategic alternative for sustainable long-term care, challenging the primacy of institutional models.

Finally, the last chapter, *Perspective Chapter: Juxtaposing the Courtesy Stigma of Mental Illness and Family Caregiver Role Strain*, examines the heavy intersection of caregiver role strain and the courtesy stigma surrounding mental illness, highlighting how social isolation and systemic neglect diminish the quality of life for those providing essential family support. It advocates for a deeper recognition of these unique challenges to better inform the development of targeted support services.

Based on the presented synthesis, these chapters delineate a clear strategic vision for the future of Long-Term Care (LTC). This vision is predicated on a fundamental reorientation of national health systems, prioritizing a deep integration with primary and community healthcare. The paramount strategic objective is twofold: to shift the axis of care from the often inadequate and costly hospital environment to the domestic and community setting, and to promote more efficient management of hospital resources. This transition allows for the liberation of inpatient beds, optimizing their use for acute and more complex cases, while simultaneously providing a more appropriate response to chronic and ongoing support needs.

The realization of this model requires the synergistic implementation of the identified pillars. The recognition and empowerment of informal caregivers, the focus on life-course prevention, and the incorporation of cultural specificities are not ends in themselves, but strategic means to underpin an integrated system. Deinstitutionalization, as a strategic shift, does not signify an absence of care but rather its provision in an environment that prioritizes comfort, autonomy, and quality of life. This well-being-centered approach, grounded in sustained basic care delivered in proximity, constitutes the cornerstone of a truly resilient, person-centered LTC system.

Thus, this work argues that overcoming the current crisis in LTC demands more than financial adjustments or demographic responses; it requires a reimagining of the very paradigm of care. The call is for a systemic transformation towards models that, while scientifically robust, are profoundly human. These models must be capable of sustaining dignity throughout life via an effective, integrated, and compassionate support network, founded on the bedrock of primary care and the comfort of home and community.

This work presents a bold, panoramic vision of Long-Term Care, challenging conventions by synthesizing the critical perspectives of leading voices worldwide. It is more than a collection of chapters; it is a roadmap for building more humane, sustainable, and equitable care systems. We encourage you to delve into its pages, confront its arguments, and help shape the transformative solutions our societies urgently need.

Wilson Abreu
ESEP, University of Porto
Porto, Portugal

Chapter 1

Introductory Chapter: Long-Term Care– Ethical Foundations, Systemic Integration, and Pathways for Change in Health and Social Care Systems

Wilson Abreu

1. Conceptual foundations of long-term care

As global populations continue to age, long-term care (LTC) has emerged as a critical pillar of contemporary health and social policy. This introduction offers a comprehensive exploration of LTC through conceptual, ethical, and systemic lenses, emphasizing foundational values such as dignity, autonomy, and cultural responsiveness. It critically examines prevailing models of care, including institutional, community-based, and integrated approaches, and evaluates their alignment with person-centered principles.

The demographic transition toward aging populations has placed long-term care (LTC) at the forefront of global health and social policy. With life expectancy rising and fertility rates declining, societies face increasing pressure to provide sustained, high-quality care for individuals experiencing chronic illness, disability, or age-related dependency. The World Health Organization (WHO) projects that by 2050, the number of people aged 60 and older will double to 2.1 billion globally [1]. This demographic shift demands not only technical and financial responses but also ethical and philosophical reflection on the value of human life and the societal obligation to care.

Over the past 10 years, we have had the opportunity to conduct research on support systems for individuals with advanced dementia and their family caregivers. Studies were carried out in collaboration with researchers and healthcare professionals from over 30 countries across five continents. The overall conclusion indicated that countries are at different stages of development regarding long-term care. Most notably, the findings indicate that the majority of these systems remain underdeveloped, poorly adapted to the demographic realities of their respective countries, and characterized by insufficient public investment, as measured by the percentage of GDP allocated to this sector.

One study explores the relationship between frailty, functional dependence, and healthcare needs among community-dwelling people with moderate to severe dementia [2]. Despite receiving structured home-care via Integrated Community Care Teams, participants – especially those with severe frailty – exhibited high levels of unmet needs in areas such as food preparation, medication management, toileting, and communication. The study highlights that even within organized LTC frameworks, care remains fragmented and insufficiently tailored to the complex realities of advanced dementia. Critically, findings suggested that current LTC models may not adequately address the intersection of frailty and dementia, underscoring the need for more responsive and flexible care strategies that reflect demographic shifts and evolving clinical demands. This calls for policy and practice reform in dementia care.

Later, another study was related to family caregiver burden and psychological distress linked to the frailty and functional dependency of a relative with advanced dementia [3]. Long-term care is addressed through the lens of community-based support. The study highlights the role of Integrated Community Care Teams in supporting dyads of dementia patients and their caregivers. Findings reveal persistent high levels of caregiver burden and psychological distress, suggesting that current long-term care provisions may be insufficient. Despite ongoing support, a large part of caregivers reported moderate or severe burden, indicating a gap between policy intentions and lived experiences. The study underscores the need for more robust, proactive long-term care strategies to sustain family caregiving and protect caregiver well-being.

LTC, as explored worldwide, is more than a set of services – it is a societal commitment to uphold dignity, autonomy, and inclusion. As [4] argue that effective long-term care systems must be fundamentally anchored in the principles of respect for individual dignity, responsiveness to evolving needs, and a person-centered approach that prioritizes the unique preferences, values, and autonomy of older adults. Only through such ethically grounded frameworks can these systems adequately address the complex and diverse requirements of aging populations.

Long-term care refers to a range of services and supports provided to individuals who need help with daily tasks or more complex activities (IADLs) over a long period. These services may be delivered in institutions (e.g., nursing homes), community settings, or private homes, and they include medical, emotional, social, and recovery-related support.

According to the World Health Organization [1], long-term care (LTC) includes a coordinated system of care activities delivered by both informal caregivers – such as family members – and trained professionals. These services are designed to support individuals experiencing a lasting decline in intrinsic capacity, helping them maintain a level of independence that aligns with their basic human rights, personal freedoms, and inherent dignity. This definition highlights the ethical imperative of care and the need for systems that respect personal independence and social inclusion.

Long-term care and palliative care overlap in their shared commitment to person-focused, dignity-preserving support, and in practice through combined service delivery for people with chronic or serious conditions. From an idea-based view, LTC and palliative care (PC) both focus on full, long-term support for people with declining health, chronic illness, or terminal conditions. Despite different main goals – recovery and maintenance in LTC versus symptom relief and emotional support in PC – both models share values of care, relationships, and respect for dignity [5]. In practice, combining LTC and PC is increasingly seen as necessary in health systems dealing with aging populations and multiple illnesses. Silva et al. [6] note that many people in LTC settings – like nursing homes or home care – develop conditions that need palliative care, such as advanced dementia, cancer, or organ failure. In these cases, PC methods are added to LTC routines, allowing for timely pain relief, planning ahead, and family support. This overlap is especially clear in elderly care, where the line between long-term and end-of-life care is often blurred.

Separation between LTC and PC services can leave needs unmet, especially in systems where palliative care is narrowly defined or lacks resources. Clear ideas and aligned policies are needed to ensure people in LTC get the right palliative care as their conditions change. As [7] notes, newer PC models support early integration, which fits well with LTC's focus on prevention and flexibility.

2. The long-term care systems worldwide: The nordic leadership

As populations age in societies, long-term care (LTC) systems face growing pressure to provide accessible, high-quality services. Following this, we offer a comparison of LTC spending across EU Member States, using country-specific laws to show structural differences. It argues that strong legal systems are essential to ensure fairness, sustainability, and readiness for demographic change.

Due to the rapid aging process, Europe and Japan have intensely problematized their Long-Term Care systems, as they face demographic pressures that are greater than those of many southern countries with younger populations. Looking at EU countries, by 2050, nearly one-third of the population will be aged 65 or older [8]. This shift increases demand for LTC services, which support people with chronic illnesses or physical limitations. National health services must adjust through smart spending and legal changes to maintain care standards and social protection.

As Europe sees more older adults – many with dementia, cancer, or other chronic conditions – the need for LTC is rising. At the same time, fewer births and smaller younger populations mean fewer family caregivers, putting more pressure on formal care systems. EU countries currently spend between 0.5% and 3.2% of GDP on LTC, with Nordic countries spending the most. National policies vary widely, affecting how care is given, paid for, and organized. Growing pressure on public health budgets, like the NHS, is worsened by the use of expensive hospital beds for people who need long-term help, not emergency care.

These systems are no longer optional – they're essential to handle rising dependency and ensure lasting, respectful care for Europe's aging population.

LTC systems in EU countries are key for:

- Supporting independence and dignity in older adults [9].
- Reducing hospital use through community-based options [10]
- Helping informal caregivers, who provide most of the care in many countries [11].
- Ensuring fairness and access, especially for vulnerable groups. [12]

Here's a look at LTC spending (% GDP) and key laws in some selected countries [13–20], [21–25]

- **Sweden**: ~ 3.2%. LTC follows the Social Services Act (2025 update), focusing on equal access and local government responsibility.

- **Netherlands**: ~ 3.0%. The Long-Term Care Act (WLZ) ensures full coverage for both home and institutional care, managed by the Care Needs Assessment Center.

- **Germany**: ~ 2.5%. The LTC Insurance Act covers all citizens; 2025 updates added more care funds and flexible budgets.

- **France**: ~ 1.9%. LTC is managed by the ALD system and regional health offices; 2025 changes aim to improve funding and expand palliative care rights.

- **Belgium**: ~ 2.0%. LTC is managed by regions; recent changes focus on reintegration and tighter benefit rules.

- **Spain**: ~ 1.1%. The Dependency Law (2006) serves as the foundation for LTC; the 2025 updates focus on reducing institutional care and expanding the workforce.

- **Poland**: ~ 0.6%. Managed by the Ministry of Family and Social Policy; LTC is still developing and lacks coordination.

The legal setup shows significant differences among countries. Countries like Sweden and the Netherlands include LTC in their welfare systems, providing access to all. Others, like Spain and Poland, are updating their systems to include informal care and reach more people. Clear laws and funding are needed to address gaps, regional differences, and staff shortages.

3. Ethical foundations and models of care

Respect for human life is a cornerstone of LTC philosophy. The principle of autonomy, the right to age with dignity, and the imperative to avoid institutional neglect are recurrent themes in the literature. Bos et al. [26] highlight the ethical imperative behind long-term care by stating that it should be seen not just as a policy area or service system, but as a deep moral responsibility carried by societies toward their most vulnerable people.

LTC systems differ widely across countries, shaped by welfare systems, cultural traditions, and historical practices. Common models include:

- Institutional care: Residential facilities offering round-the-clock support, often for people with high needs.

- Home-based care: Services provided in the person's home, including nursing, personal care, and recovery support.

- Community-based care: Day centers, short-term relief care, and social support that help people stay in their homes.

- Informal care: Unpaid care provided by family or friends, often without official recognition or assistance.

Barreira et al. [27] describe a basic framework for LTC systems, identifying three connected ideas: continuity of care, cross-sectoral integration, and personalization. These are key to building care plans that are clear, flexible, and suited to each person. Continuity means support continues over time and through changes in health or living situations; integration helps connect medical, social, and community services; and personalization focuses on adjusting care to match each person's needs and values. The authors warn that fragmentation between services weakens LTC, emphasizing that the fragmentation of services undermines the very essence of LTC, which is to provide seamless, person-centered support across time and settings.

Scott et al. [28] identify a series of ongoing and connected problems that especially limit access to long-term care (LTC) services for minority groups. One of the biggest challenges is language mismatch, which seriously affects both the admission process and the quality of care – especially for recent immigrants and people from language minority backgrounds. Cultural incongruence makes access to and quality of care more difficult. Many older adults from minority backgrounds prefer care settings that match their cultural habits, such as food choices, religious practices, and social traditions. When LTC services don't meet these needs, people may feel isolated, less healthy, and unwilling to use available services. These systems must recognize and support the different cultural, language, and social backgrounds of those receiving care. As [28] point out, the challenge is to balance consistent care with the need for personalized support that reflects each person's background. With global demand for LTC growing, it's more important than ever to design policies that not only recognize but actively support ethnic diversity. This includes offering high-quality care at home, where cultural comfort and personal independence can be better maintained.

4. Challenges and future research priorities

Despite the growing body of literature on LTC, significant research challenges persist, particularly in understanding and addressing disparities in access and outcomes. These challenges are compounded when considering minority populations, whose experiences are shaped by intersecting factors such as race, ethnicity, language, migration status, gender identity, and socio-economic position.

The review by [28] identifies major methodological weaknesses limiting the reliability of long-term care (LTC) research, especially for minority populations. Significant heterogeneity in study designs prevents comparable analyses and hinders generalizable conclusions. Many studies lack adjusted statistical models, reducing validity by failing to account for key confounders. Qualitative depth is also insufficient, offering limited insight into minority elders' lived experiences and cultural expectations. The authors call for intersectional, participatory, and culturally sensitive research approaches that meaningfully involve minority communities. Future work should evaluate targeted interventions, compare international systems, and use longitudinal designs to track evolving trends. Without more rigorous, inclusive research, disparities in LTC access and outcomes will persist, undermining equity and quality of care.

Long-term care is a multidimensional challenge that connects with ethics, policy, culture, and economics. As populations age and become more diverse, national health and social care systems must change to ensure dignity, fairness, and inclusion for everyone who needs long-term support. The way LTC is integrated into national systems varies widely across countries, reflecting different welfare models, government structures, and cultural values. Yet, common problems remain: fragmentation, underfunding, staff shortages, and inequitable access.

Paying for LTC is still a difficult and unsettled issue. In many places, LTC receives less funding than hospital care, even though it's becoming more important. Public support varies, with some countries relying heavily on personal payments or income-based benefits, which increase inequality and hinder access. The question of who should pay – individuals, families, insurance companies, or governments – is not just technical but deeply political, reflecting choices about fairness, shared risk, and justice between generations.

Given these challenges, LTC systems must explore new paths. This doesn't mean giving up core values but rethinking them for today's world. Several new ideas are emerging, each with significant impacts.

Governments must find solutions that fit their own societies. Change can start locally. One direction is to connect care across different services. Gaps between health, social, and housing services hurt continuity and personal care. Joined-up care models – like case managers, shared budgets, or team-based approaches – try to fix this. Digital tools, such as shared health records, remote monitoring, and AI support, can help but must be used carefully, respecting privacy and digital skills.

Another promising direction is to grow community and home-based care. Most older adults prefer to stay at home, and it's often cheaper and better for their independence. However, it requires strong support systems, such as safe housing, transport, short-term relief for caregivers, and training. Shared housing, mixed-age living, and age-friendly cities are part of this, challenging traditional ideas of care homes.

A third direction is to rethink the role of families and communities. While unpaid care shouldn't be taken for granted, policies can better support those who provide it. This includes pay, legal rights, flexible jobs, and emotional support. At the same time, community involvement and volunteering can build care networks beyond family ties. These models require cultural change and strong support, but they offer strength and deeper relationships.

Finally, new ideas must come with responsibility and open discussion, as expected in democratic societies. The future of LTC is not just a technical issue but a social decision. Leaders, professionals, researchers, and citizens must talk openly about values, priorities, and trade-offs. Pilot programs, policy trials, and learning from other countries can help but must be tested carefully and openly. The WHO (2022) [29] highlights that strengthening community-based and long-term care (LTC) services can significantly reduce avoidable hospital and emergency-department use. When older adults or people with chronic conditions receive timely support at home or in community settings, deterioration and crises are less frequent. Investing in LTC prevents unnecessary long hospital stays for patients who primarily need social or functional support rather than acute care. This shift improves care quality, reduces pressure on hospitals, and helps rebalance costs across the National Health Service by allocating resources to more efficient, person-centered services that maintain independence and prevent institutional overuse.

In short, aging and caregiver shortages are not isolated problems but symptoms of wider transformations in population, work, family, and welfare systems. Long-term care (LTC) must, therefore, respond not with minor adjustments but with bold, value-driven, and research-based reforms. Integrated care, community support, caregiver protection, rights-based approaches, and shared leadership are not idealistic ambitions – they are necessary directions that require investment, creativity, and strong institutions. These challenges are substantial, but they also offer an opportunity to build care systems that are fair, compassionate, and resilient for future generations. Addressing them demands a commitment to ethical principles, better coordination, and culturally sensitive practices, supported by research grounded in real-life experiences and diverse perspectives.

Long-term care encompasses a wide range of important matters that shape its development, implementation, and future direction. Among these are matters involving the preparation, training, and continuous development of staff, including the relevance of learning modalities, skill acquisition, and competencies that support care for individuals with complex needs. There are also important matters connected to the design of policies, procedures, and service pathways that guide communication, coordination, and overall care experiences.

Another set of matters relates to the organization of long-term care across home, community, and primary healthcare settings, including the alignment of these environments with cultural preferences and structural capacities. The circumstances of family caregivers present further important matters, including those associated with the multiple responsibilities they balance, the financial and employment implications of their role, and the broader impact on family wellbeing. Matters linked to caregiver burden, emotional strain, and the need for supportive interventions also stand out, affecting quality of life and care provision.

Finally, the development of coherent conceptual models, adequate state investment, and sustainable organizational structures emerges as an overarching matter that determines the functionality, continuity, and effectiveness of long-term care systems. One aspect to note is what emerges in countries that, in demographic terms, have very young populations. Studies systematically appear that attempt to problematize conceptual and operational perspectives of long-term care (LTC), adopting a proactive approach to preparing for the future.

This book brings together a broad set of LTC situations from different societies and cultural contexts, all united by a concern for how effectively care systems support people.

Acknowledgement

The author acknowledges the use of AI tools for language checks.

Author details

Wilson Abreu
ESEP, University of Porto, Porto, Portugal

*Address all correspondence to: wjabreu@esenf.pt

References

[1] World Health Organization. State of Long-term Care: Conceptual Framework for Assessment and Continuous Learning in Long-term Care Systems. Copenhagen. 2024. Available from: https://www.who.int/europe/publications/i/item/WHO-EURO-2024-10363-50135-75508

[2] Abreu W, Tolson D, Jackson GA, Staines H, Costa N. The relationship between frailty, functional dependence, and healthcare needs among community-dwelling people with moderate to severe dementia. New Jersey: Health Soc Care Community. 2019;**27**(3):642-653. DOI: 10.1111/hsc.12678

[3] Abreu W, Tolson D, Jackson G, Costa N. A cross sectional study of family caregiver burden and psychological distress linked to frailty and functional dependency of a relative with advanced dementia. London: Dementia: the international journal of social research and practice. 2018;**1**:1

[4] Kringos DS, Bos VLLC, Poldrugovac M, Wammes JD, Barbazza E, Ivanković D, Merten H, MacNeil Vroomen JL, Klazinga NS. Performance indicators on long-term care for older people in 43 high- and middle-income countries. BMC Health Services Research. 2025;**25**:Article 460. Available from: https://bmchealthservres.biomedcentral.com/articles/10.1186/s12913-025-12573-4

[5] Bertaud S, Wilkinson D, Kelley M. The heart of palliative care is relational: A scoping review of the ethics of care in palliative medicine. BMC Palliative Care. 2025;**24**(150). DOI: 10.1186/s12904-025-01784-5

[6] Silva DAA, Machado GRR, da Silva BG. Relationship Established between the Concepts of Palliative Care and Long-term Care: An Integrative Review. São José dos Pinhais, Brazil: Home Publishing; 2023. DOI: 10.56238/homeII sevenhealth-117

[7] Yang X, Chen X, Liu Q, Yao L. A brief literature review of conceptual models in palliative care. In: Bollig G, Zelko E, editors. Palliative Care – Current Practice and Future Perspectives. London: IntechOpen; 2024. DOI: 10.5772/intechopen.1003782

[8] European Commission. Long-term Care Report: Trends, Challenges and Opportunities in an Ageing Society. Vol. **II**. Brussels: Country profiles, Publications Office; 2021a, 2021. Available from: https://data.europa.eu/doi/10.2767/183997

[9] Eurocarers. National Reports on the Implementation of the Council Recommendation on Access to High-quality Long-Term Care. Brussels, Belgium, 2024

[10] Thapa BB, Li X, Galárraga O. Impacts of community-based care program on health care utilization and cost. American Journal of Managed Care. 2022;**28**(4):187–191. PMID: 35420747. DOI: 10.37765/ajmc.2022.88862

[11] CARES Project. Benchmark report on social care sectors at the national and EU level. CARES Project No. 2024-1-RO01-KA220-ADU-000251559. Brussels: Eurocarers; 2025

[12] European Commission. Healthcare and Long-term Care Workforce:

Demographic Challenges and Potential Contribution of Migration and Digital Technology. Brussels: Publications Office of the EU; 2021. Available from: https://op.europa.eu/en/publication-detail/-/publication/de896328-771b-11eb-9ac9-01aa75ed71a1/language-en

[13] European Commission. Poland Long-Term Care Implementation Reports. 2024. Available from: https://commission.europa.eu/publications/implementation-reports-2024_en

[14] European Commission. Romania LTC Implementation Report. 2024b. Available from: https://commission.europa.eu/publications/implementation-reports-2024_en

[15] Asensio Vázquez M, García Ciria C, López Molina G. Funcas. Spain's Long-term Care System at a Crossroads: Demographic Pressures and Workforce Challenges. 2025. Available from: https://www.funcas.es/articulos/spains-long-term-care-system-at-a-crossroads-demographic-pressures-and-workforce-challenges/

[16] Government of Sweden. Preventive, Accessible and Knowledge-based Social Services. 2025. Available from: https://www.government.se/articles/2025/03/preventive-accessible-and-knowledge-based-social-services/

[17] Government.nl. Long-term Care Act (WLZ). - Bundesministerium Für Gesundheit. (2025). Pflegeversicherung.). 2025. Available from: https://www.government.nl/topics/nursing-homes-and-residential-care/long-term-care-act-wlz

[18] IGAS & IGF. Structural Reform of France's LTC System. Paris. 2024

[19] Rothgang H, Müller R, Unger R. Long-term care in Germany: Between social insurance and demographic pressure. Health Policy. 2024;**128**(3):345–358

[20] Sowa-Kofta A, Badora-Musiał K. Long-term care in Poland: Challenges and policy directions. European Journal of Social Policy. 2024;**34**(2):210–225

[21] World Bank. Romania's Way Forward in LTC. Technical Inputs to the 2023-2030 LTC Strategy. Bucharest: International Bank for Reconstruction and Development; 2022

[22] World Bank. Strategic Review of Long-Term Care Services in Poland. International Bank for Reconstruction and Development; 2025. Available from: https://hdl.handle.net/10986/43111

[23] Tsutsui T. Japan's long-term care insurance system: Achievements and challenges after two decades. International Journal of Health Planning and Management. 2024;**39**(1):1–15

[24] Vabo SI. The Territorial Dimension of Long-Term Care for Older People. In: Kazepov Y, editor. Rescaling Social Policies towards Multilevel Governance in Europe: Social Assistance, Activation and Care for Older People. London: Routledge; 2017. DOI: 10.4324/9781315244433-9

[25] Szebehely M, Meagher G. Nordic eldercare: Weak universalism becoming weaker? Journal of European Social Policy. 2024;**34**(1):45–60

[26] Bos VLLC, Poldrugovac M, Wammes JD, Barbazza E, Ivanković D, Merten H, MacNeil Vroomen JL, Klazinga NS, Kringos DS. Performance indicators on long-term care for older

people in 43 high- and middle-income countries. BMC Health Services Research. 2025;**25**. Article 460. Available from: https://bmchealthservres.biomedcentral.com/articles/10.1186/s12913-025-12573-4

[27] Barreira LF, Paiva A, Araújo B, Campos MJ. Challenges to Systems of Long-Term Care: Mapping of the Central Concepts from an Umbrella Review. International Journal of Environmental Research and Public Health. 2023;**20**:1698. DOI: 10.3390/ijerph20031698

[28] Scott MM, Mayhew A, Jeong A, Shaver N, Lapenskie J, Hsu AT, Tanjong-Ghogomu E, Tanuseputro P, Huang E, Welch V. Access to long-term care for minority populations: A systematic review. Canadian Journal on Aging/La Revue Canadienne du Vieillissement. 2022;**41**(4):577–592. DOI: 10.1017/S0714980822000046

[29] WHO. Rebuilding for sustainability and resilience: strengthening the integrated delivery of long-term care in the European region. 2022. Copenhagen: WHO Regional Office for Europe Available from: https://iris.who.int/server/api/core/bitstreams/69795ee0-d42f-4af2-889a-dd9c5b439af1/content

[30] Abreu W, Tolson D, Jackson GA, Staines H, Costa N. The relationship between frailty, functional dependence, and healthcare needs among community-dwelling people with moderate to severe dementia. Health & Social Care in the Community. 2019;**27**(3):642–653. Epub 2018 Nov 7. PMID: 30402986. DOI: 10.1111/hsc.12678

[31] Torres S. Ethnicity and old age: Toward a contextualized understanding of ethnic minority aging in Europe. Journal of Aging Studies. 2019;**49**: 1–9. DOI: 10.1016/j.jaging.2019.100772

Chapter 2

Perspective Chapter: Family Caregivers – Pioneering Pathways in Long-Term Care Innovation and Research

Fatma Abdalla Mohamed Abdalla

Abstract

This chapter explores how caregivers, as non-professional caregivers – often family members – play a critical role in daily disease management, and their understanding of prevention strategies directly impacts patient outcomes. The chapter presents findings from a recent study assessing caregiver awareness, attitudes, and educational needs. It also highlights gaps in caregiver training and proposes community-based educational interventions tailored to cultural and socioeconomic contexts. By framing the topic within the broader context of long-term care for chronic illnesses, this chapter underscores the importance of caregiver empowerment through inclusive policy practices and targeted research, which are essential to reducing healthcare burdens and improving the quality of life for patients and families.

Keywords: caregivers, pioneering, pathway, long-term, care

1. Introduction

1.1 The concept of caregivers

Kleinman states that care is the human glue that binds communities, societies, and families together [1]. Caregivers are operationally defined as those responsible for the ongoing physical care and emotional support of individuals who are unable to care for themselves [2]. Care can be organized in either a formal or informal manner [3]. In an informal setting, care is provided by a person's friends or family. Volunteers and family members play a vital role in the process of caring for individuals with disabilities or chronic illnesses [4].

1.2 The demand for caregivers

Due to the aging population in Europe, the demand for informal care is expected to rise [5]. According to a study conducted by Verbakel et al. (2017), the estimated number of informal caregivers in Europe could range from 10% to 25% of the overall population [6].

1.3 The role of caregivers

The role of caregiving varies depending on the situation, cause, and type of disability. The trajectory begins with the caregiver recognizing that something is wrong with the care recipient. This often involves taking the individual to medical appointments and communicating with their healthcare provider. The trajectory continues to intensify as the need for care increases. This includes hiring care providers, monitoring the patient's medications, managing their symptoms, and providing emotional support. Caregivers then need to complete self-care tasks such as dressing, managing insurance, addressing symptoms, and assisting with chores. Depending on the situation, end-of-life care can involve placing the patient in a nursing home or a hospice program. The trajectory indicates that the tasks for the caregiver are cumulative. As the need for care increases, the role of caregiving becomes stressful, more complex, and time-consuming [7].

There are multiple activities and tasks associated with caregiving. Caregivers engage in interpersonal and cognitive processes that involve problem-solving, monitoring the well-being of their loved ones, and communicating with others. This includes maintaining their social connections and advocating for their loved ones' health and medical care. The tasks that a caregiver completes depend on their skills, health status, values, and preferences, as well as other factors such as the availability of resources and the quality of their relationship with the recipient [8].

Although family involvement in medical and nursing tasks has existed for a long time, it has become more complex and prevalent. As a result, more elderly individuals are now being cared for at home instead of in nursing homes or hospitals [9].

This often involves interacting with complex medical devices. The shift in the role of the caregiver is attributed to the reduction in hospital admissions and the increasing complexity of treatment options for acute and chronic conditions in non-institutional settings [7].

2. Family caregiver support for patient self-management during chronic, life-limiting illness

The daily activities of patients with illnesses are referred to as self-management. It involves managing their symptoms, treatments, lifestyle modifications, and the spiritual, cultural, and psychosocial effects of their illness [10].

The novel themes revolved around the family caregiver's role in supporting their loved ones with chronic and life-limiting illnesses. They included focusing on the patient's needs, activating resources to help the family caregiver, and supporting the patient living with a chronic and life-limiting illness. The various factors that influence the support family caregivers provide for their loved ones with chronic and severe illnesses were identified. These factors included the patient's health status, personal and environmental characteristics, and available resources. The role of the family caregiver in supporting patient self-management is complex and involves multiple processes [11].

When a family member is involved in the management of a sick loved one's illness, the term "self and family-management" is often used to refer to the individual's daily activities. This indicates that patients are managing their conditions with the help of their caregivers [12].

Substantial evidence indicates that there are effective interventions that assist family members in providing the necessary support and care for their sick loved ones. However, these evidence-based studies did not focus on the specific needs and challenges of family caregivers of people with chronic and life-limiting illnesses [11].

3. Impact of caregiving

The effects of caregiving can be both highly individualized and wide-ranged. Caregivers are at a higher risk of experiencing negative impacts in various aspects of their lives, such as their health, economic security, and quality of life [7].

Strong evidence shows that family members who look after older adults are at risk, as they are more prone to experiencing emotional distress, depression, and anxiety than non-caregivers. Furthermore, caregivers reportedly have lower self-ratings, elevated cortisol levels, and are more prone to experiencing chronic diseases. The various factors that affect the quality of life for caregivers can also contribute to their negative outcomes. These include the intensity of their caregiving, the lack of choice in their role, and the perception of the suffering of the recipient. The physical and social functioning of the caregiver, as well as the support they receive, are also factors that can contribute to these negative effects. Caregivers who shift from a low-intensity role to a high-intensity one experience more adverse effects [8].

In addition, they may benefit from providing care. Being able to provide care to a loved one can help instill confidence in the caregiver, make them feel closer to the recipient, and ensure that the recipient is receiving the best possible care. However, the exact effects of this type of support can vary depending on the individual's contextual and personal characteristics [7].

The body of evidence on the negative effects of providing care is far greater than that on the positive effects. This is because researchers have been conducting studies to identify individuals who are at risk of experiencing these effects and to assess the public health consequences of this type of support [8]. Documenting these effects is a vital first step in developing effective interventions and policies to help caregivers [7].

4. Well-being and quality of life

The psychological and mental states of caregivers are affected by the loss of their autonomy and the demands of their patients. The quality of life of caregivers is significantly affected [13–15]. Besides the quality of life, the psychological well-being of caregivers is also impacted by the stress levels they experience. Some of the factors that can influence this are the ways in which they cope with the burden of caring for their patients [16–18].

5. Emotional stress and psychological stress

Caregivers experience emotional stress differently from psychological distress due to their duties. The stress process is affected by various factors, including the types of stressors they encounter, their subjective appraisal of these stressors, and their resources, which can act as protective factors [19–21].

6. Anxiety and depression

The caregivers tend to have higher levels of anxiety and depressive symptoms. These conditions affect their ability to perform their daily tasks and make it hard to maintain their motivation. Depression is a type of psychological disorder that affects people's behavior and emotions. It can be triggered by negative self-evaluation [13, 14, 22].

7. Burden associated with caregiving

The burden of caregiving is defined by Zarit et al. as the damage caused by providing care for a loved one, which can affect physical and emotional health, economic conditions, and social life. There are two components to this concept: subjective overload and the emotional response to caregiving. According to Zarit and colleagues, subjective overload is a psychological feeling associated with caregiving. On the contrary, the objective burden refers to the type of burden the primary caregiver bears to provide the best possible care for their loved one. It is linked to the various tasks and challenges the caregiver must face regularly [23].

Women are more likely to provide care for dependent people than men [24]. This has been known to result in a decline in physical and mental health and a higher burden of care for women. In addition, being a male caregiver and receiving external help are associated with a lower caregiving burden [25–27]. This has been positively linked to caregiver satisfaction and alleviation of the caregiving burden [28].

8. Other problems associated with caregiving

Many informal caregivers face challenges in managing their own lives and coping with emotions [29]. Being a caregiver has a significant impact on the well-being of those who provide care. Substantial evidence reveals that this situation negatively affects the financial well-being of caregivers. They often must leave their jobs to care for these individuals due to the high demands placed on them, making it difficult to reconcile their work and family lives [21, 23, 30–35]. This can lead to financial problems stemming from the costs of providing care for a disabled individual. One study showed that when financial barriers were reduced, caregivers were more likely to experience improved well-being [21]. Many caregivers feel that their role as a family member has shifted to that of a caregiver due to the stress and other factors they encounter while providing care [36].

9. Assessing and addressing family caregivers' needs and risks

The identification of the needs and risks of caregivers is a complex issue. To effectively integrate the use of standardized assessment tools into the practice of healthcare, a variety of factors must be considered. Current practices lack consistency when it comes to identifying the needs and risks of caregivers. This issue is often addressed by various indirect and direct approaches. According to participants, the use of a standardized assessment could help improve the quality of care for patients and enhance communication between clinicians and caregivers. Various barriers prevent the use of a standardized caregiver assessment, such as time and reimbursement issues, liability concerns, a lack of awareness, and challenges regarding the autonomy of patients. To help facilitate the uptake of this practice, participants suggested that the use of self-administered tools be paired with post-screen discussions with practitioners [37].

Instead of using standardized tools to assess the needs and risks of caregivers, primary care physicians utilize informal, unstructured discussions to gather information. There are varying types of referrals and topics discussed. Evidence indicates that there is a lack of translation of caregivers' assessments between research and practice [38].

10. Defining caregiver needs: Balancing subjectivity

Although the perception of caregivers in identifying needs is often regarded as the primary factor influencing the identification of needs, it is not always the sole basis for making decisions regarding the services required. In addition to the caregiver's perception, other factors, such as the availability of resources and the cost of services, are also considered to determine the appropriate program for addressing the needs of individuals. This is because, in both social and health care, it is essential to understand what services are needed to prevent harm and how they are delivered [39].

There is a lot of evidence indicating that there are unmet needs among individuals with dementia, which are linked to various factors such as psychological distress and a lack of daytime activities. These issues contribute to the poor social health of the individuals. Most informal caregivers also reportedly have inadequate information about the disease's trajectory, post-diagnostic care, and home support. On the contrary, formal caregivers reportedly have related information needs [40].

11. Caregiver competency and training needs

A survey on caregiver competency and training needs was conducted. Compared to the external observers, caregivers were more likely to assess themselves higher in various aspects of their job performance. For instance, they were more likely to say that they are capable of recording and reporting information, understanding major illnesses, and ensuring safety and infection control. Both external observers and caregivers agreed that it is important for caregivers to undergo training. They preferred to receive one to two hours of additional training every year. The difference between the assessments of caregivers by external observers and their self-evaluations was significant. This suggests that training and re-training of caregivers are needed [41].

12. Individual and protective factors

Even though the impact of providing care is immense, many factors can help protect the well-being and health of caregivers. According to studies, the quality of life for caregivers improves significantly if they have a good relationship with their patients [42] and a supportive network [43]. They also possess positive personality traits that help them cope with their environment. Having a greater level of collaboration and agreement between two caregivers can enhance their effectiveness and involvement. Addressing certain health-related conflicts can also improve the capacity of caregivers to support older individuals [44].

Social support can help buffer stress, which is a common factor that can affect the health and well-being of patients. It can also influence the different processes of illness and the treatment of these conditions. One of the most important factors that caregivers must consider is their self-esteem. Having a positive personality trait can help them cope well with the stressful situations they have to face. Low self-esteem can lead to a cycle of reluctance to ask for assistance and restricted social connections, which can worsen the caregiver's burden. However, having a strong self-esteem can help caregivers manage their stress levels. Resilient self-esteem can also help caregivers reduce their anxiety and improve their quality of life when dealing with stressful situations. Being resilient is also linked to the effectiveness of caregiving. It can help a caregiver maintain a positive quality of life and avoid experiencing negative effects from their actions. Caregivers who felt secure in their decision-making abilities and did not feel pressured were more satisfied with their lives [45]. Evidence suggests that a multidisciplinary team, supported through welfare systems, should be created to support caregivers [29].

13. Knowledge, attitude, and practices of caregivers

Although most caregivers possess a good understanding of the disease, those who care for individuals with dementia often exhibit a negative attitude toward it. The findings of this study indicate that a comprehensive evaluation of the attitudes and knowledge of these caregivers is necessary to improve the quality of care for both the patients and the caregivers [46].

Lack of awareness regarding the use of aerosol therapy and controller medications is a major issue that affects the quality of life for people with asthma. In addition, children with asthma often do not receive enough nutritious food. This is why community groups must develop effective strategies to raise awareness about the disease [47].

Evidence revealed that most caregivers have inadequate knowledge and practice when it comes to providing for older individuals. This review provides valuable insight into the needs and knowledge of family caregivers. It recommends that further studies be conducted on the contextual factors affecting the care of older adults to identify effective solutions and improve the knowledge, practice, and support for family caregivers. The knowledge and practice of family caregivers regarding the care of older individuals are not satisfactory in several study settings. This review identified various needs of family caregivers, such as access to information about the activities of the elderly, training from healthcare professionals, financial issues, health services, and legal concerns. The lack of support for family caregivers has been identified as a major issue that affects the quality of life of older individuals. This review recommends that further studies be conducted on the various needs of family caregivers. These studies should also identify effective ways to improve their knowledge and practice [48].

The evidence suggests that there is a need for regular educational programs for caregivers of people with epilepsy. This study can help develop effective resources for those who are looking after their loved ones [49].

The knowledge gap regarding epilepsy among caregivers has been identified. This issue can be addressed by improving the attitudes and practices of those who look after children with epilepsy to enhance the overall quality of life for children with epilepsy [50].

Family members and caregivers must take the necessary steps to improve their attitudes toward their loved ones with Alzheimer's disease. This can be achieved through various psychosocial interventions and referrals to the appropriate Alzheimer's associations [51].

14. Coping and adjustment in caregivers

14.1 Use of problem- versus emotion-focused coping

Compared to non-caregivers, caregivers relied less on positive strategies and used problem-focused coping. These types of coping methods are known to be more adaptive and reduce psychological distress [52].

Several studies have shown that caregivers use problem-focused strategies to reduce their burden [53]. Some of these strategies include reducing their work hours, using paid help, taking advantage of social support, and integrating care into their daily routines. They also accept financial hardship and incorporate care into family culture. Other problem-focused coping strategies involve acting or modifying behavior in the client's surroundings to reduce labor and time spent. These can include dealing with the client's physical limitations, managing their health, communicating with them, and finding humor [53–58].

According to Williams et al., in 2014, problem-focused methods involved conversing with others and reviewing the health conditions of the client to gain a greater sense of control [58].

15. Use of cognitive strategies

Some cognitive strategies focused on the perception of the caregiver's role. Caregivers reported that appreciating the caregiver's role and its benefits, finding meaning in their experiences, and maintaining autonomy helped them adapt to the situation [59–61].

Caregivers reported that reframing their experiences helped them cope with their situation. They also found humor in their expressions when they were feeling helpless. Some people who chose to view their caregiving as a voluntary act of compassion stated that adopting a gain mentality instead of a loss mentality was beneficial [61].

16. Factors associated with psychological adjustment

Numerous factors can be linked to psychological adjustment. Social support is known to be associated with positive adjustment, as it can help reduce distress and improve the health of caregivers [62, 63].

In 2015, Wong et al. found that a strong and positive relationship between the caregiver and their spouse was associated with positive adjustment [64]. In addition, regular positive social interactions were regarded as vital factors that could help promote resilience and adjustment [56, 65, 66].

According to the caregivers, social opportunities that allow them to share information and experiences positively affect their outcomes and adjustment [55, 56].

17. Harmonizing caregiver needs assessment across service settings, countries, and cultures

The various sectors of the health and social care industry are often characterized by their institutional boundaries, which makes it difficult to bridge these gaps, especially in countries with large and diverse populations. They also lack coordinated funding streams and national health systems. In countries with small and socially cohesive populations, such as Denmark, the public is responsible for providing a safety net for older adults. However, in developed countries, this responsibility is often unevenly distributed and underfunded. The main gaps in the assessment of the needs of older adults stem from the perception of the private sector as primarily responsible for providing care. This can affect the expectations of caregivers and their willingness to provide information about their needs. In addition, when needs are assessed using measures developed in other languages, the translation of the information cannot be considered fully comparable to that of the target group. To improve the assessment of the needs of older adults, a cross-cultural collaboration is needed. This can help create a framework for developing effective and efficient tools and methods. The goal of the assessment is to provide the best possible care and support to individuals with dementia and their caregivers [67].

18. The effect of the family-centered empowerment model

Individuals caring for a loved one suffering from multiple sclerosis are at risk of experiencing care burden, which can negatively affect their quality of life. The goal of this study is to determine the effects of family-centered empowerment model (FCEM) on the caregiver's care burden. The results of the study revealed that all demographic attributes were homogeneous. Before the intervention, there had been no significant difference between the two groups concerning the mean score of care burden. The repeated measures test also did not reveal any significant interaction between the two groups in terms of time and treatment. The effects of the FCEM on alleviating the care burden were not significant. It is important to keep in mind the various factors that affect the intervention's impact on the care burden [68].

19. Family caregivers' processes to support patient self-management

The family caregiver's process in supporting their loved one with a chronic and life-limiting illness includes focusing on the patient's needs, activating resources to assist them, and helping them live with a chronic, life-limiting illness.

20. Focusing on the patient's illness needs

The goal of the process is to provide family members with the necessary skills and responsibilities to help their loved ones manage their illness. This process involves learning about the patient's health condition and developing strategies to support their self-management. In addition to learning about the patient's illness, family caregivers can also provide the patient with the necessary support. Through this process, family members can gain essential information about their loved ones' health conditions. They can also learn the skills they can use to support their loved ones [69–72].

According to the article's authors, various aspects of the support process are involved in the care of patients. Some of these include being able to encourage the patient's emotional and physical health, acting as a patient advocate, and providing practical help with household chores [11].

The activities of family caregivers vary depending on the patient's ability and willingness to manage their health conditions. For instance, the activities of a family caregiver may be focused on helping the patient manage their health conditions, or they may be involved in other aspects of the support process. The patient's health condition, the type of care they are receiving, and the value of their resources all play a role in the development of the partnership between the patient and the caregiver. The concept of focusing on the needs of patients refers to various types of partnerships between family members and patients. For instance, one of the partners may assist the patient with scheduling an appointment or perform other tasks on their behalf, whereas the other partner may provide the patient with minimal support [11].

21. Activating resources to support oneself as a family caregiver

The concept of activating resources to support oneself as a family caregiver is a process that involves the utilization of various resources to help the individual maintain and improve their role in patient management [11]. Various resources are reflected in psychosocial [73–75] and spiritual domains [76]. Some of the skills and tasks that family caregivers can perform when they activate resources include praying, seeking emotional support, and utilizing respite care. Family caregivers can vary in the extent to which they use their resources depending on the needs of their patients over time. According to Williams and colleagues, family caregivers need to activate their resources to sustain their caregiving duties. They noted that those who utilized multiple self-care techniques coped well with the emotional and physical challenges of caring for a loved one [76].

22. Supporting a patient living with a chronic, life-limiting illness

The process of supporting a patient living with a chronic, life-limiting illness involves various skills and tasks, such as managing one's own emotions, addressing the physical health of the patient, and making sense of being a caregiver. Family caregivers also have to address the high emotional burden that they carry [11].

In 2015, Applebaum et al. published a study showing how physical and emotional issues affect the well-being of family caregivers. It highlighted the overlapping responsibilities of managing one's physical and emotional health [77].

Some of the tensions that family members experience when it comes to supporting their patients revolve around balancing their own health needs with supporting the patients' needs versus advocating on the patient's behalf. They suggest that this type of support should be prioritized. Caregivers experience a wide range of emotions when it comes to supporting their patients [11].

Clinicians also play a vital role in supporting family caregivers in making informed decisions regarding their health. They should assess the various aspects of the family caregiver's role and provide them with the necessary resources to improve their quality of life [78].

Family caregivers should be referred to mental health experts to enhance their stress management, coping capacity, and overall quality of life. Case management, government support, and comprehensive care provided by specialists and health professionals can help them manage their own mental and emotional well-being. An effective intervention for family caregivers should be developed. Family caregiver-specific components should be included in multi-component interventions designed to improve the self-management of patients. The intervention program must be carried out properly. It should involve an initial assessment designed to identify the multiple skills needed to improve their well-being. In addition to the usual multi-component interventions, it is also important that the approach be expanded to include other types of interventions aimed at improving the self-management of patients [11].

Author details

Fatma Abdalla Mohamed Abdalla
Department of Nursing, College of Nursing and Health Sciences, Jazan University, Jazan, Saudi Arabia

*Address all correspondence to: fatimaabdalla008@gmail.com

References

[1] Kleinman A. The soul of care: The moral education of a husband and a doctor. New York: Penguin; 2020. Available from: https://cdn.penguin.co.uk/dam-assets/books/9780141992419/9780141992419-sample.pdf [Accessed: 2025-October-24]

[2] Mohamed, F.A. et al. Caregivers' knowledge and attitude toward the preventive measures of sickle cell crisis related to their socio-demographic characteristics. Rawal Medical Journal. 2025;**50**. Available from: https://www.ejmanager.com/mnstemps/27/27-1729193219.pdf?t=1761323254 [Accessed: 2025-October-24]

[3] Albin B, Siwertsson C, Svensson JO. Informal care of the elderly in Sweden-carers' situation. Aotearoa New Zealand Social Work. 2011;**23**(1/2):66–77

[4] Roth DL, Fredman L, Haley WE. Informal caregiving and its impact on health: A reappraisal from population-based studies. The Gerontologist. 2015;**55**(2):309–319

[5] D'Agostino A, Ghellini G, Navarro M, Sánchez A. Overview of the Quality of Life in Europe. In: Analysis of Socio-Economic Conditions, 1st Edition. London: Publications Office of the European Union; 2021: 362. DOI: 10.4324/9781003053712

[6] Verbakel E, Tamlagsrønning S, Winstone L, Fjær EL, Eikemo TA. Informal care in Europe: Findings from the European Social Survey (2014) special module on the social determinants of health. The European Journal of Public Health. 2017;**27**(suppl_1):90–95

[7] Schulz R, Beach SR, Czaja SJ, Martire LM, Monin JK. Family caregiving for older adults. Annual Review of Psychology. 2020;**71**(1):635–659

[8] Eden J, Schulz R, editors. Families Caring for an Aging America. National Academies of Sciences, Engineering, and Medicine. Washington, DC: Natl. Acad. Press; 2016. DOI: 10.17226/23606.

[9] Reinhard SC, Feinberg LF. The escalating complexity of family caregiving: Meeting the challenge. In: Family Caregiving in the New Normal. Elsevier: Academic Press; 2015. p. 291–303. Available from: https://www.sciencedirect.com/book/9780124170469/family-caregiving-in-the-new-normal [Accessed: 2025- October-24]

[10] Richard AA, Shea K. Delineation of self-care and associated concepts. Journal of Nursing Scholarship. 2011;**43**(3):255–264

[11] Schulman-Green D, Feder SL, Dionne-Odom JN, Batten J, En Long VJ, Harris Y, Wilpers A, Wong T, Whittemore R. Family caregiver support of patient self-management during chronic, life-limiting illness: A qualitative metasynthesis. Journal of Family Nursing. 2021;**27**(1):55–72

[12] Grey M, Knafl K, McCorkle R. A framework for the study of self- and family management of chronic conditions. Nursing Outlook. 2006;**54**(5):278–286

[13] Darragh AR, Sommerich CM, Lavender SA, Tanner KJ, Vogel K, Campo M. Musculoskeletal discomfort, physical demand, and caregiving activities in informal caregivers. Journal

of Applied Gerontology. 2015;**34**(6):734–760

[14] Hussain R, Wark S, Dillon G, Ryan P. Self-reported physical and mental health of Australian carers: A cross-sectional study. BMJ Open. 2016;**6**(9):1–10. Available from: https://bmjopen.bmj.com/content/bmjopen/6/9/e011417.full.pdf

[15] Kuorinka I, Jonsson B, Kilbom A, Vinterberg H, Biering-Sørensen F, Andersson G, Jørgensen K. Standardised Nordic questionnaires for the analysis of musculoskeletal symptoms. Applied Ergonomics. 1987;**18**(3):233–237

[16] Bambara JK, Turner AP, Williams RM, Haselkorn JK. Social support and depressive symptoms among caregivers of veterans with multiple sclerosis. Rehabilitation Psychology. 2014;**59**(2):230

[17] McKeown LP, Porter-Armstrong AP, Baxter GD. The needs and experiences of caregivers of individuals with multiple sclerosis: A systematic review. Clinical Rehabilitation. 2003;**17**(3):234–248

[18] Borren I, Tambs K, Idstad M, Ask H, Sundet JM. Psychological distress and subjective well-being in partners of somatically ill or physically disabled: The Nord-Trøndelag Health Study. Scandinavian Journal of Psychology. 2012;**53**(6):475–482

[19] Alshammari SA, Alzahrani AA, Alabduljabbar KA, Aldaghri AA, Alhusainy YA, Khan MA, Alshuwaier RA, Kariz IN. The burden perceived by informal caregivers of the elderly in Saudi Arabia. Journal of Family and Community Medicine. 2017;**24**(3):145–150

[20] Bramble RJ, Duerk EK, Baltes BB. Finding the nuance in eldercare measurement: Latent profiles of eldercare characteristics. Journal of Business and Psychology. 2020;**35**(1):29–43

[21] Alfaro N, Lázaro P, Gabriele G, Garcia-Vicuña R, Já J, Sevilla J. Perceptions, attitudes and experiences of family caregivers of patients with musculoskeletal diseases: A qualitative approach. Reumatología Clínica (English Edition). 2013;**9**(6):334–339

[22] Polenick CA, DePasquale N. Predictors of secondary role strains among spousal caregivers of older adults with functional disability. The Gerontologist. 2019;**59**(3):486–498

[23] Zarit SH, Reever KE, Bach-Peterson J. Relatives of the impaired elderly: Correlates of feelings of burden. The Gerontologist. 1980;**20**(6):649–655

[24] Amabile TM, Gryskiewicz ND. The creative environment scales: Work environment inventory. Creativity Research Journal. 1989;**2**(4):231–253

[25] Katbamna S, Ahmad W, Bhakta P, Baker R, Parker G. Do they look after their own? Informal support for South Asian carers. Health and Social Care in the Community. 2004;**12**(5):398–406

[26] Kurauchi G, Endo M, Odaira K, Ono R, Koseki A, Goto M, Sato Y, Kon S, Watanabe N, Sugawara N, Kimura E. Caregiver burden and related factors among caregivers of patients with myotonic dystrophy type 1. Journal of Neuromuscular Diseases. 2019;**6**(4):527–536

[27] McCusker J, Latimer E, Cole M, Ciampi A, Sewitch M. Major depression

among medically ill elders contributes to sustained poor mental health in their informal caregivers. Age and Ageing. 2007;**36**(4):400–406

[28] Tough H, Brinkhof MW, Siegrist J, Fekete C. Subjective caregiver burden and caregiver satisfaction: The role of partner relationship quality and reciprocity. Archives of Physical Medicine and Rehabilitation. 2017;**98**(10):2042–2051

[29] Akgun-Citak E, Attepe-Ozden S, Vaskelyte A, van Bruchem-visser Rl, Pompili S, Kav S, Acar S, Aksoydan E, Altintas A, Aytar A, Baskici C. Challenges and needs of informal caregivers in elderly care: Qualitative research in four European countries, the TRACE project. Archives of Gerontology and Geriatrics. 2020;**87**:103971. DOI: 10.1016/j.archger.2019.103971

[30] Elliott TR, Berry JW, Richards JS, Shewchuk RM. Resilience in the initial year of caregiving for a family member with a traumatic spinal cord injury. Journal of Consulting and Clinical Psychology. 2014;**82**(6):1072

[31] Secinti E, Selcuk B, Harma M. Personal and familial predictors of depressive feelings in people with orthopedic disability. Health Psychology Report. 2017;**5**(3):227–239

[32] Dreer LE, Elliott TR, Shewchuk R, Berry JW, Rivera P. Family caregivers of persons with spinal cord injury: Predicting caregivers at risk for probable depression. Rehabilitation Psychology. 2007;**52**(3):351

[33] Ryff CD. Happiness is everything, or is it? Explorations on the meaning of psychological well-being. Journal of Personality and Social Psychology. 1989;**57**(6):1069

[34] Beck AT, Epstein N, Brown G, Steer RA. An inventory for measuring clinical anxiety: Psychometric properties. Journal of Consulting and Clinical Psychology. 1988;**56**(6):893

[35] Thrush A, Hyder A. The neglected burden of caregiving in low- and middle-income countries. Disability and Health Journal. 2014;**7**(3):262–272

[36] Rodger D, Neill MO, Nugent L. Informal carers' experiences of caring for older adults at home: A phenomenological study. British Journal of Community Nursing. 2015;**20**(6):280–285

[37] Riffin C, Wolff JL, Estill M, Prabhu S, Pillemer KA. Caregiver needs assessment in primary care: Views of clinicians, staff, patients, and caregivers. Journal of the American Geriatrics Society. 2020;**68**(6):1262–1270

[38] Riffin C, Wolff JL, Pillemer KA. Assessing and Addressing Family Caregivers' Needs and Risks in Primary Care. Journal of the American Geriatrics Society. 2021;**69**(2):432–440

[39] Marosszeky N, Rix MD, Owen AG. Knowing what you need to know about needs assessment. National Health Outcomes Conference Wollongong, Australia: Australian Health Outcomes Collaboration 2006

[40] Koh WQ, Roes M, de Vugt M, Szegin D, Gonçalves-Pereira M, Müller N, Diaz A, Casey D, Ingram C, Walden AK, and Thyrian JR. What are the unmet needs in people affected by dementia? A scoping review of reviews. Aging and Mental Health. 2025;1–20. DOI: 10.1080/13607863.2025.2534406

[41] Lee DY, Lee SB, Lim KM, Choi YJ, Kang DY. Survey on caregiver

competency and retraining needs. Public Health Nursing. 2024;**41**(6):1265–1270

[42] Torgé CJ.Freedom and imperative: Mutual care between older spouses with physical disabilities. Journal of Family Nursing. 2014;**20**(2):204–225

[43] Pierce GR, IG S, BR S. General and relationship-based perceptions of social support: Are two constructs better than one? Journal of Personality and Social Psychology. 1991;**61**(6):1028

[44] Russell AM, Bonham M, Lovett R, Pack A, Wolf MS, O'Conor R. Characterizing caregiver roles and conflict in health management support to older people with multiple chronic conditions. Journal of Applied Gerontology. 2024; **43**(4):386–395

[45] Cejalvo E, Marti-Vilar M, Merino-Soto C, Aguirre-Morales MT. Caregiving role and psychosocial and individual factors: A systematic review. InHealthcare. 2021;**9**(12):1690

[46] Parveen S, Mehra A, Kumar K, Grover S. Knowledge and attitude of caregivers of people with dementia. Geriatrics & Gerontology International. 2022;**22**(1):19–25

[47] Awan AS, Munir SS.Asthmatic children: Knowledge, attitude and practices among caregivers. The Professional Medical Journal. 2015;**22** (01):130–136

[48] Ab Ghani NN, Makhtar A, Elias SM, Ahmad N, Ludin SM. Knowledge, practice and needs of caregiver in the care of older people: A review. International Journal of Care Scholars. 2022;**5**(3):70–78

[49] El-Amin RO, El-Sadig SM, and Mohamed IN. Knowledge, attitudes, and practices of caregivers of children with epilepsy in Sudan. Epilepsy & Behavior. 2021;**123**:108283. DOI: 10.1016/j.yebeh.2021.108283

[50] Negussie AS, Dehan MF, Mekonnen SA, Zelleke TG. Knowledge, attitudes, and practices of caregivers with children diagnosed with epilepsy attending a pediatric outpatient clinic: A descriptive, cross-sectional, questionnaire-based study in Addis Ababa, Ethiopia. BMC Neurology. 2024;**24**(1):252

[51] Khalil A, Aladwani N, Aljehani S. Relationship between knowledge, attitude, and burden among Alzheimer's family caregivers in Jeddah, Saudi Arabia. Saudi Journal of Nursing and Health Care. 2020;**3**:167–174

[52] Mausbach BT, Chattillion EA, Roepke SK, Patterson TL, Grant I. A Comparison of Psychosocial Outcomes in Elderly Alzheimer Caregivers and Noncaregivers. The American Journal of Geriatric Psychiatry. 2013;**21**(1):5–13.

[53] Hawken T, Turner-Cobb J, and Barnett J. Coping and adjustment in caregivers: A systematic review. Health Psychology Open. 2018;**5**(2): 2055102918810659. DOI: 10.1177/2055102918810659

[54] Dickson A, O'Brien G, Ward R, Flowers P, Allan D, O'Carroll R. Adjustment and coping in spousal caregivers following a traumatic spinal cord injury: An interpretative phenomenological analysis. Journal of Health Psychology. 2012;**17**(2):247–257

[55] Kita M, Ito K. The caregiving process of the family unit caring for a frail older family member at home: A grounded theory study. International

Journal of Older People Nursing. 2013;**8**(2):149–158

[56] McCausland Kurz J, Cavanaugh JC. A qualitative study of stress and coping strategies used by well spouses of lung transplant candidates. Families, Systems, & Health. 2001;**19**(2):181

[57] Sun F.Caregiving stress and coping: A thematic analysis of Chinese family caregivers of persons with dementia. Dementia. 2014;**13**(6):803–818

[58] Williams KL, Morrison V, Robinson CA. Exploring caregiving experiences: Caregiver coping and making sense of illness. Aging and Mental Health. 2014;**18**(5):600–609

[59] Kitter B, Sharman R. Caregivers' support needs and factors promoting resiliency after brain injury. Brain Injury. 2015;**29**(9):1082–1093

[60] Thornton N, Hopp FP."So I Just Took Over": African American Daughters Caregiving for Parents with Heart Failure. Families in Society. 2011;**92**(2):211–217

[61] Zegwaard MI, Aartsen MJ, Grypdonck MH, Cuijpers P. Differences in impact of long term caregiving for mentally ill older adults on the daily life of informal caregivers: A qualitative study. BMC Psychiatry. 2013;**13**(1):103

[62] Haley WE, Roth DL, Coleton MI, Ford GR, West CA, Colllins RP, Isobe TL. Appraisal, coping, and social support as mediators of well-being in black and white family caregivers of patients with Alzheimer's disease. Journal of Consulting and Clinical Psychology. 1996;**64**(1):121

[63] Pakenham KI, Bursnall S. Relations between social support, appraisal and coping and both positive and negative outcomes for children of a parent with multiple sclerosis and comparisons with children of healthy parents. Clinical Rehabilitation. 2006;**20**(8):709–723

[64] Wong OL, Kwong PS, Ho CK, Chow SM, Kwok T, Wong B, Ho V, Lau A, Ho F. Living with dementia: An exploratory study of caregiving in a Chinese family context. Social Work in Health Care. 2015;**54**(8):758–776

[65] Kaplan RL. Caregiving mothers of children with impairments: Coping and support in Russia. Disability & Society. 2010;**25**(6):715–729

[66] Ruiz-Robledillo N, De Andrés-García S, Pérez-Blasco J, González-Bono E, Moya-Albiol L. Highly resilient coping entails better perceived health, high social support and low morning cortisol levels in parents of children with autism spectrum disorder. Research in Developmental Disabilities. 2014;**35**(3):686–695

[67] Borson S. Assessing caregiver needs. International Psychogeriatrics. 2021;**33**(4):331–334

[68] Mousaei FM, Mirhosseini S, Mafi MH, Günaydın N, Zendehtalab HR. Effect of support based on family centered empowerment model on care burden in family caregivers of patients with multiple sclerosis. Frontiers in Public Health. 2023;**11**:1115311

[69] Fujinami R, Otis-Green S, Klein L, Sidhu R, and Ferrell B. Quality of life of family caregivers: Challenges faced in care of the lung cancer patient. Clinical Journal of Oncology Nursing. 2012;**16**(6):E210

[70] Pappa K, Doty T, Taff SD, Kniepmann K, Foster ER. Self-management program participation and social support in Parkinson's disease: Mixed methods evaluation. Physical & Occupational Therapy in Geriatrics. 2017;**35**(2):81–98

[71] Retrum JH, Nowels CT, Bekelman DB. Patient and caregiver congruence: The importance of dyads in heart failure care. Journal of Cardiovascular Nursing. 2013;**28**(2): 129–136

[72] Dikkers MF, Dunning T, Savage S. Information needs of family carers of people with diabetes at the end of life: A literature review. Journal of Palliative Medicine. 2013;**16**(12): 1617–1623

[73] Gysels MH, Higginson IJ. Caring for a person in advanced illness and suffering from breathlessness at home: Threats and resources. Palliative and Supportive Care. 2009;**7**(2):153–162

[74] Keesing S, Rosenwax L. Is occupation missing from occupational therapy in palliative care? Australian Occupational Therapy Journal. 2011;**58** (5):329–336

[75] Holden RJ, Schubert CC, Mickelson RS. The patient work system: An analysis of self-care performance barriers among elderly heart failure patients and their informal caregivers. Applied Ergonomics. 2015;**47**:133–150

[76] Williams A, Duggleby W, Eby J, Cooper RD, Hallstrom LK, Holtslander L, Thomas R. Hope against hope: Exploring the hopes and challenges of rural female caregivers of persons with advanced cancer. BMC Palliative Care. 2013;**12**(1):44

[77] Breitbart W, and Masterson M. Meaning-centered psychotherapy in the oncology and palliative care settings. In: Russo, Netzer, Stefan, Schulenberg, Alexander, Batthyány. Clinical Perspectives on Meaning: Positive and Existential Psychotherapy. Cham: Springer International Publishing; 2016. p. 245–260

[78] International Family Nursing Association. IFNA position paper on generalist competencies for family nursing practice [Internet]. 2015

Chapter 3

Global Burden of Lifestyle Diseases and Pressure Injuries: Nutritional Predictors and Impact on Family Health Outcomes

Donnette A. Wright, Natoya Wade and Audra T. Williams

Abstract

The elderly population is among a special group of the population classified as vulnerable due to their susceptibility to disease and disorder as well as their financial and physical dependence of other segments among the population. This group of individuals is at risk of chronic non-communicable diseases, lifestyle diseases, and other public health concern pressure injuries. This disorder is a group of health conditions including bed sores, decubitus ulcers, and pressure sores. Individuals who are vulnerable are at greater risk of being diagnosed and afflicted with the condition. Mobility, nutritional status, and general health (concomitant) disease modify the risk profile of the population. The paradox of longevity increased disability is pronounced in the current public health landscape especially concerning pressure injury status. The impact of aging and health outcomes impairs social functioning and burdens the dynamics of the family unit often resulting in caregiver role strain. The role of the healthcare team in preventing and responding to ill-health and the resulting impact is paramount among the aging population. The resultant recommendations of active screening, primary health care, health education, nutritional support, and social support are the critical strategies to improve the health outcomes of this vulnerable population toward morbidity profile and healthcare outcomes among the elderly. This chapter explores the current evidence, incidence, contributory factors, and public health recommendations for best practice of healthcare among the aging population.

Keywords: pressure injury, nutritional predictor, family outcome, lifestyle disease, nutritional status

1. Introduction

In the public health sphere, pressure injuries (PIs), also known as pressure ulcers or decubitus ulcers, are described as localized damage to skin and the soft tissues below usually occurring over bony prominence or where a medical device is worn [1]. They constitute a major concern, undermining the quality of life, and increasing morbidity and mortality, and contributes extensive financial burden to patients and the healthcare system. Although mostly preventable, PIs vastly affect hospitalized patients, specifically those with the restricted mobility and chronic non-communicable diseases, whether in the acute or in the long-term care facilities [2]. The World Health Organization predicts that the aging population is expected to reach 426 million between the years 2020 and 2050, with pressure ulcers being a concern for this vulnerable population. Older adults, with a PI, are usually plagued by other comorbidities such as fluid and electrolyte disorders, diabetes mellitus, nutritional disorders, and dementia, contributing to a more complex healing process [3]. Varied advancements in medicine and wound care management have improved patient outcomes with multimodal adjuvant therapies for prevention and treatment; however, this problem still exists. According to the National Pressure Injury Advisory Panel (NPIAP), pressure injuries can occur over skin or underlying tissues, usually over a bony prominence or related to medical devices, as a result of pressure, friction, shear, moisture, or any combination of these factors [4]. PIs differ according to its severity of tissue loss and wound bed characteristics, which lend itself to a NPAUP classification system for staging [5]. Preventing and managing PIs require a multidisciplinary approach focusing on the underlying issues in combination with other associated risk factors. Malnutrition, sometimes undiagnosed, has played a role in prolonging the healing process. There is a direct proportional relationship between malnutrition and PI development and impaired wound healing. Evidence supports adequate dietary inclusion of calorie (energy), protein, zinc, Vitamin A, C, D, and specific amino acids such as arginine and glutamine, which positively impacts tissue repair and collagen synthesis and being essential for wound healing [6]. The presence of a PI has the potential to disrupt one's quality of life due to chronic or cyclic pain associated with the disease process, body image disturbance, odor and drainage, prolonged hospitalization for treatment, and management of complications. Structure and psychosocial roles within the family can be grossly affected, contributing to an overwhelming emotional and financial burden as well as caregiver burnout [7]. The current evidence provides data that the elderly population is expanding significantly, and they are vulnerable and at risk of lifestyle diseases and pressure injuries. This chapter will elucidate the nature of PIs, its global impact, the nutritional factors that promote efficient treatment of the disease, the impact PIs have on immediate family members, and the coping mechanisms that families employ to mitigate its effects. The chapter will also offer recommendations for the best practice in health promotion and care for optimal health outcomes among the aging population.

2. Global burden of pressure injuries

The incidence of PIs continues to grow despite increased medical knowledge, advances in technology, and wound care management [8]. The global prevalence of pressure injuries is estimated to be 3.17 million based on analysis of the 2019 GBD analysis with 481,423 DALYs [9, 10]. The development of PIs adversely affects approximately 12% of hospitalized patients with over 50% being categorized as stage I and stage II pressure injuries [9, 10]. Prevalence may vary based on setting, as patients with spinal cord injuries report a higher prevalence rate of 44% [11]. In acute care facilities in the USA alone, approximately 2.5 million patients per year suffer from

PIs [12]. Prior studies on PIs have tended to focus on hospital based and ICU settings, whereas patients in community, home care, and age care facility settings are often overlooked. The true prevalence of PIs is therefore under-estimated.

Treatment cost associated with PIs has risen exponentially, with PIs being ranked as 3rd in terms of economic burden, preceded by cancer and cardiovascular diseases. A recent NPIAP study reported an annual cost of 3.6B, with other studies concluding a greater economic burden of 26.8B annually [13, 14]. Studies have indicated that the cost associated with preventing PIs is substantial when compared to that for treatment [15]. When compared to other chronic diseases, PI, a type of chronic wound, has a two to six times higher mortality rate with annual deaths amounting to 60, 000 [16].

Older adults aged >60 have a greater prevalence rate of PI than the younger age group across the various levels of sociodemographic index (SDI). There has been a worrying trend of age standardized rate (ASR) deaths among the older age groups with individuals between 80 and 84 having an ASR of death of 7.21 when compared to those >95 showed an accelerated rate of up to 51.72 [17]. Regions with higher SDI documented reduced ASRs as opposed to an increase in ASRs reported in low middle and low SDI. The ASR of Disability adjusted life years (DALY) globally continues to grow among the older age group >60 (up to 20.65) with exponential burden in individual aged 95 and older (322.25–485.2); however, ASRs of DALY in low SDI were the highest across all age groups, notable with older adults>95 with 820.33 [17].

3. Risk factors

Pressure injury development is a notable concern for patients, family members, caregivers, and members of the health care team. Intrinsic and extrinsic factors have been attributable to the development of PIs and it is of vital importance that a thorough understanding is reached in order to effectively manage the underlying cause. Intrinsic factors include nutritional deficits, advanced age, low blood pressures, fever, and smoking. Extrinsic factors are pressure (intensity of pressure, duration of pressure, tissue tolerance), shear, friction, moisture associated with urinary or fecal incontinence [9, 17, 18].

3.1 Nutrition and PI

Nutrition is the most important factor stimulating normal cellular function such as tissue repair and regeneration. Adequate nutritional support is essential for all patients; however, patients with a PI or at risk for PI development require optimized support in preventing further skin breakdown and to facilitate the healing process [19]. Malnutrition, both macro- and micronutrient forms, is a type of nutritional debilitation that is linked to the development of PI in patients along the age continuum, but more so in the aging population. Macronutrients such as carbohydrate, protein, fats as well as fluids and micronutrients including vitamins and minerals all have a critical role in the maintaining optimal skin integrity and promoting wound healing. *Dehydration, reduced energy intake, and low protein consumption are attributable to rapid skin breakdown when coupled with other risk factors such as pressure, friction, shear, and moisture*. Approximately 1.5–2.1 g of protein may be loss in wound exudate per day and as such emphasis must be placed on preventing further depletion as well as dehydration [20]. Determining nutritional status is multifaceted. There is no specific laboratory test to confirm malnutrition; however, levels of serum proteins such as albumin, pre-albumin, transferrin, and retinol-binding protein are frequently used as biochemical indicators of malnutrition [21]. Other biochemical markers including triglycerides, CRP, zinc, copper, and cytokines provide insight into the nutritional status of at risk and diagnosed PI patients. In addition to serum proteins, anthropometric measurements such as height, weight and body mass index (BMI) are used [22].

Weight loss in the last 6 months	
<5%	**Mild loss**
5–10%	Moderate loss
>10%	Severe loss
Body mass index (BMI)	
<18.5 kg/m2	Underweight
18.5–24.9 kg/m2	Normal weight
25.0–29.9 kg/m2	Overweight
≥30 kg/m2	Obese
<90% ideal body weight	Malnourished

Adapted from Evans [22].

Box 1. *Weight indicators for malnutrition.*

3.2 Healing-related nutritional needs

The presence of a wound increases the body's metabolic demand for nutrients. The phases of wound healing are supported by various nutrients for adequate and timely wound closure, thus reducing the risk of complications [23]. Malnutrition is a strong contributor of adverse events such as the development of new wounds, PIs, and diminished quality of life, as well as other lifestyle diseases. Judicious screening for malnutritional risk at admission and at the first sign of change in patient's condition is key for early diagnosis and swift intervention [24].

Nutritional support is dependent on multiple factors including age, gender, weight, height, BMI, activity level, and current comorbidities. With protein and fluid depletion from the wound each day, an increase in nutrients is needed to support the metabolic and physiological needs to prevent progression and promote healing [25].

Caloric need requirement ranges from 20 to 35 kcalories per kg body weight per day. In the presence of a wound or an injury, the body's caloric need for adults increases to 30-35kcalories/kg body weight for patients with PI or those at risk of PI with malnutrition risk [4, 26]. Yamamoto et al. [27] highlighted a correlation between energy intake and pressure ulcer healing.

Post-injury, the body's need for protein increases exponentially, with the recommended daily allowance (RDA) of protein being approximately 1.25–1.5 g per kilogram per day, while in a healthy person, the recommended daily allowance of protein is 0.8–1 g per kilogram body weight per 24 hours [4, 28].

Proteins are composed of building blocks essential and non-essential amino-acids and are necessary for the tissue repair and regeneration and collagen synthesis [28].

Impaired amino-acid balance can negatively affect wound healing process resulting in delayed wound healing especially at the inflammatory, proliferation, and remodeling phases of healing [29]. Increase in protein stores aides in collagen synthesis and epithelialization that are indicative of positive signs for advanced healing.

Arginine and glutamine have been well documented in the recent years to have substantial effects on wound healing. An essential amino acid, arginine stimulates the release of growth hormone and also insulin-like growth factor I (IGF-I), which improves wound healing [19]. Reports indicate its effect on inflammatory response, collagen synthesis, and wound contraction [30]. Arginine supplementation with other nutrients may be beneficial in improving wound healing outcome [31, 32].

One of the most abundant amino acids in the body, glutamine has immunomodulatory and anti-inflammatory effects. Glutamine requirement of 0.3–0.4 g per kilogram per day is recommended in patients with wounds [28]. Supplementation of other vitamins and minerals has shown to be efficacious in wound healing including selenium, zinc, and vitamins A, C, E which support epithelialization, tissue oxygenation, and inflammatory response and other physiological recovery processes in wound healing [33].

4. Impact of PIs on the family

Pressure injuries commonly affect older adults (>60) and have been seen to contribute to psychological, physical, and social disruptions to immediate and extended family members [34]. Caregivers of people who suffer from chronic illnesses have been primarily family members, this is due to the expensive nature of nursing homes, and the perceived lack of care caused by an overburden health system at public facilities and are considered instrumental in caring for chronic patients [35]. Family members who offer or are pressured into the role of caregiver are generally female, married, have low levels/basic education, and have low-paying jobs [7, 36, 37]. It is of interest that these characteristics of caregivers except for being married share similar characteristics with those who are found in vulnerable populations. Though caregivers and patients can be good support for each other, they can ultimately be a source of stress [7], and the constant attention that patients with PIs need tends to consume the life of the caregiver which significantly contributes to the burden that the caregivers feel and ultimately to the global healthcare system [35].

The phrase burden of care is commonly found in the literature that deals with chronic patients and can be defined as the level of strain that a carer perceives from caring for a chronically ill, disabled, or an aged family member or a loved one [35]. It also negatively correlates with quality of life, in that, the more a caregiver feels burdened by the care that they provide is the poorer they perceive their quality of life. Psychological predictors of burden of care include stressors, anxiety about caring, feelings of sadness, guilt, and helplessness [7] while negative predictors include upper middle education or higher, strong social support networks, and how well the family functions despite the chronically ill loved one [37]. These feelings can stem from seeing their loved one in a state of decline [7] regardless of the carer's sex [36, 37]. The lack of knowledge that caregivers have about treating PIs can also impact their psychological well-being. Knowing when PIs are developing and seeking trained professionals to provide support can be overwhelming. In addition, taking anecdotal information from people who are not trained health practitioners can cause the worsening of the loved one's wounds, which then contributes to feelings of guilt [7].

This is exacerbated by the caregivers' feelings of moral responsibility stemming from their desire to compensate the loved one for their past absence or a debt of gratitude. This desire is evident in close knit intergenerational relationships [7].

Psychological effects of the burden of disease also stem from the lack of familial support that is given to primary caregivers [36]. Having to constantly be at the side of an ailing individual can wary the caregiver and can contribute to irritability and feelings of overwhelm that can be directed at the loved one who requires care or other family members that are not engaged directly in caring for the loved one. Support when given were mostly offered to female caregivers [36], which can act as an influencing factor to them handing over the responsibility of care to another female member of the family. First time carers for patients with PIs can encounter stress due to the unfamiliarity of the disease [7]. This lack of experience can hinder the prevention of the injury and its recovery as factors such as diet, food preparation and feeding assistance, hygiene maintenance, repositioning and use of supportive devices, and medication and dressing application are the important aspects of efficiently care for PIs [7].

The financial burden of care can stem from the lack of educational attainment of the caregivers, the reduction or loss of gainful employment due to the needs of the chronically ill loved one, and the medical costs that are associated with chronic illness. This inability to garner professional medical care is to the detriment of the loved one [7]. Few primary caregivers receive any kind of stipend from other relatives [36], which increases the psychological burden of disease. This lack of finances significantly impacts both the diet of the caregiver and the chronically ill loved one and can lead to the worsening of the loved one's condition. This will incur additional expenses that increase anxiety, depression, and stress. This cyclical process can continue for weeks, years, and even decades and will hinder the recovery of the loved one [36]. The financial burden also incorporates the lack of resources that the caregivers can extend to themselves, which will negatively impact how they function as caregivers [36]. The lack of resources may result in self-blame which often co-ocur with, or secondary to, feelings of grief and helplessness [7].

5. Coping mechanisms that families employ to mitigate the effects of PIs

Primary caregivers often do not know current practices and evidence-based pressure injury management, as such, there is an urgent need for health practitioners to provide efficient and comprehensive guidance in how to manage the PIs, namely in dressing selection and decompressing products [7]. When primary carers are equipped with the knowledge that is needed to properly care for their loved ones then recovery can take place, which would significantly impact the psychological, physical, and financial standing of not only the caregiver but also the extended family. Providing this as well as nutritional support can increase the confidence of a caregiver to hand over temporarily the care of the loved one to engage in self-care activities. This engagement in self-care activity can improve their well-being [37], which inevitably decreases feelings of overwhelm, anxiety, and depression.

6. Nutritional predictors and family health outcomes

Poor nutrient consumption may lead to adverse health outcomes such as cardiovascular diseases, diabetes, hypertension, obesity, and PI development. Family health

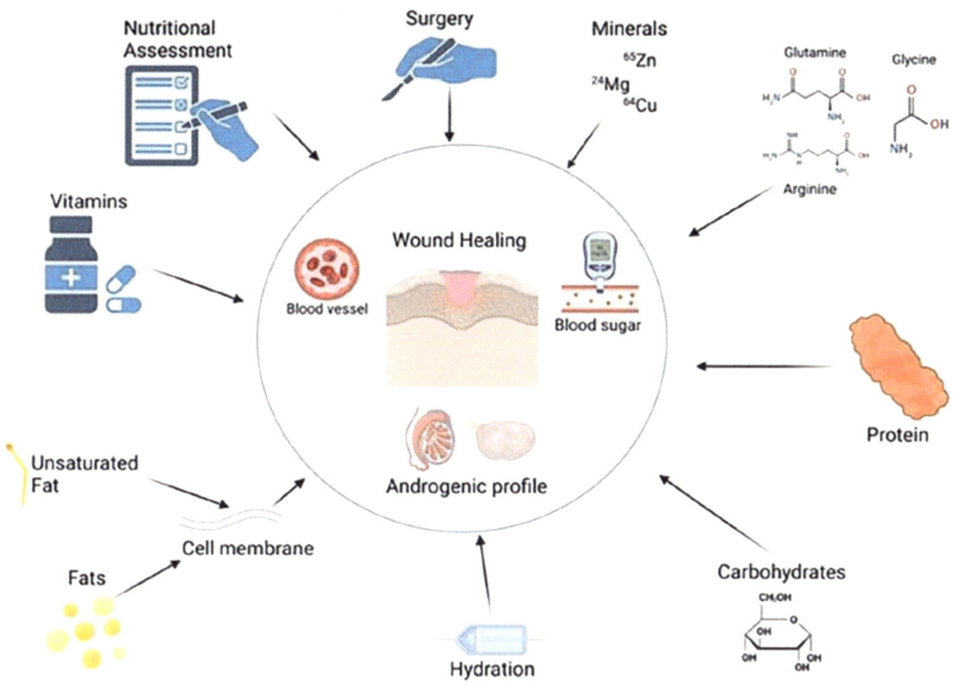

Figure 1.
Factors that potentially influence wound healing and esthetic outcomes. This is an open access article under the CC BY license. http://creativecommons.org/licenses/by/4.0/.

and well-being can be affected significantly by poor dietary intake throughout the life cycle at different stages of development, impacting individuals, family units, the community, and to a greater extent, the nation [38]. Adopting healthy eating habits and an increased level of physical activity in childhood should be fostered, as this helps to mitigate against malnutrition-associated conditions such as impaired cognition and stunted growth [39]. There are many lifestyle diseases that are linked to poor eating habits, which predominantly begin at the level of the family unit.

Effective management of PIs requires a multidisciplinary approach focusing on the underlying causative factors. PIs can be caused by a single factor or a combination and efforts must be placed on addressing these factors. Nutritional support is crucial in achieving closure of the wounds as most elderly patients might have poor nutritional status that is oftentimes undiagnosed. Comprehensive wound assessment, individualized interventions utilizing evidence-based practice with optimal wound bed preparation, appropriate dressing, and support surface selection are a key to improve the patients' outcome. In addition to nutritional support and wound management, focus must be geared toward the 'whole' individual providing a holistic approach to management (**Figure 1**).

7. Discussion: The current status of the global burden on diseases and PI among the elderly - Nutritional predictors and family outcomes

The North American population of elderly people is currently estimated at greater than half (56%) of their total population and reflects as similar ratio in international population [40]. The WHO and other organizations have projected that the population will continue to expand and has also classified this group as the fastest growing set of people [41]. An overwhelming expanse of literature presents evidence concerning the vulnerability of the aging population presenting a paradox of longevity juxtaposed with the increased disability. There are several determinants cited as promulgating the risk of disease and disorder among this segment of the population including poor knowledge, access to primary healthcare, poor knowledge, social and financial reliance, food and nutritional requirements, and physiological changes in the elderly. These factors correlate with the increased risk of physical disabilities including pressure injury. Other studies suggest that there is a feminization of the elderly where disproportionately more women are older when compared to men [42]. There is further evidence that women have greater health seeking behaviors and are less vulnerable to pressure injuries when compared to men, which provides some evidence of resilience among this sub-segment of the elderly population and forms part of the recommendations that increasing health seeking behaviors may serve as a protective factor in the development of PIs among the elderly. The evidence also suggests that increased independence and conduct of Activities of Daily Living occur in community-based elderly people [42]. This activity increases mobility and reduces bed dependence, which further reduces the susceptibility to pressure injuries among community dwelling individuals and repositioning, moisture control, and pressure redistribution inversely correlated with pressure injury [43]. Nutrition has been closely associated with pressure injuries and overall health status of all peoples and the elderly in particular [44]. Nutrition currently exists as a factor that modifies health outcomes and is directly associated with the variable. In the elderly, it has been described as generally suboptimal with the associated negative outcomes. Some evidence proposes that individuals with good biological and biochemical markers of nutrition have greater resilience and associated lower risk of pressure injuries. The data suggests that replete macronutrient and micronutrient states promote optimal biochemical status and are associated with the lower risk of PI among the elderly and all populations. This suggests that while nutritional status is generally poor or at risk of deficiency among the elderly targeted strategies to promote nutritional wellness may provide a protective effect among hospitalized as well as community dwelling elderly [45].

The physiological needs of the elderly are well documented and promoted for care and intervention and less value is place on the psychosocial status of the aging population especially family and social groups. The literature clearly represents the impact of disease and disorder on these processes describing them as stressed and strained especially as the disease and disorder burden is long term. That presents only the negative psychosocial impact aging. There is also resilience promoted through strong family and social support of the elderly with respect to the development and promotion of PIs. Strong carer support has been identified as a positive social determinant in the recovery from PIs among both hospitalized and community dwelling elderly [46]. The financial and physical wound care support promotes comprehensive response and quicker healing. This also suggests the groups of elderly with stronger family support and less susceptible to pressure injuries when compared to those with limited support.

8. Recommendations

The elderly population and the aging process present a conundrum for public health. Longevity serves as a strong positive outcome of health promotion but health care workers must be cautious in interpreting and celebrating increased life expectancy as older adults are plagued with a wide range of health risks among them lifestyle diseases and pressure injuries which are partly due to increased vulnerability. The healthcare team must be prepared for the next five decades and beyond, which provides a predictive model that forecasts a ballooning elderly population with the increased needs relative to their dependence. The evidence that underlines their vulnerability must be transformed to provide robust guidance to strengthen their future health outcomes. These recommendations include but are not limited to:

1. Regular health screenings—general physical health accessing skin integrity, biochemical markers, and nutritional status. This is designed to detect early deviations and guide strong individualized plans for health promotion and recovery [44, 47]

2. Multidisciplinary individualized health care plan—The elderly is a dynamic population with physical and physiological needs—a general care physician make essential but gerontologists, homecare assistants, dietitians, phlebotomists, social workers, and physiotherapists are important for assessing and strategically support the management of specialized deficits in the elderly

3. Individualized nutrition care support—early, targeted, and personalized nutrition support predicated on health promotion and primary care interventions is uniquely position to prevent sub-optimal nutritional states and ensure that Recommended Dietary Allowances are met in accordance with patient preferences so that nutrition serves as positive risk modifier in the development of lifestyle and pressure injuries.

4. Wound care and assessment—early and continuous skin assessment is essential for detecting early changes integrity and determining primary strategies to prevent deterioration. Community-based and secondary level comprehensive care are critical in reducing disability adjusted life years and morbidity among the elderly.

5. Promoting independence, mobility, and ADL participation—mobility has been singularly described as an inversely related factor in the determined pressure injuries. Families, communities, and the healthcare team must be trained and supported to encourage and support mobility, independence, and ADL completion among the elderly institutionalized and free dwelling individuals

6. Psychosocial and family support—carers must be guided with respect to promoting financial resilience, social competence, and physiological care to the elderly people they relate to. These factors when protected will serve as a protective factor in the development of pressure ulcers and lifestyle diseases. Similar value must be accorded to psychosocial support as with physical support as the future of health outcome elderly population is promoted in order to promote the best status.

9. Conclusion

The population of elderly people has been growing and is expected to expand in the next two decades. Their associate healthcare burden is expanding consistent with their incidence of chronic non-communicable diseases and pressure injuries. Social and physiological factors such as age, comorbidity, and nutritional status predict the healthcare risk, recovery, and overall outcome. Family units also impact the nutritional status of the elderly and their health outcomes impact the functionality of the unit. The cyclical link between nutrition, wound development, recovery, and the family unit creates a unique multimodal responsibility on the health care system—primary secondary and tertiary to support the prevention, treatment, recovery, and coping with pressure injuries in the elderly population. These processes are best supported by comprehensive screening and assessment, health education, individualized nutritional and clinical support, and specialized referral and panoptic follow-up.

Author details

Donnette A. Wright*, Natoya Wade and Audra T. Williams
The University of the West Indies, Mona, Jamaica

*Address all correspondence to: donnette.wright02@uwimona.edu.jm

References

[1] Mondragon N, Zito PM. Pressure Injury. PubMed: StatPearls Publishing; 2024. Available from: https://www.ncbi.nlm.nih.gov/books/NBK557868/

[2] Black JM, Edsberg LE, Baharestani MM, Langemo D, Goldberg M, McNichol L, et al. Pressure ulcers: Avoidable or unavoidable? Results of the National Pressure Ulcer Advisory Panel Consensus Conference. PubMed. 2011;**57**(2):24-37. Available from: https://pubmed.ncbi.nlm.nih.gov/21350270

[3] Russo CA, Steiner C, Spector W. Hospitalizations Related to Pressure Ulcers among Adults 18 Years and Older, 2006. Agency for Healthcare Research and Quality; 2008. pp. 1-9. Available from: https://europepmc.org/books/NBK54557

[4] National Pressure Ulcer Advisory Panel and European Pressure Ulcer Advisory Panel. Prevention and Treatment of Pressure Ulcer: Clinical Practice Guideline. Washington, DC: National Pressure Ulcer Advisory Panel; 2009

[5] Edsberg LE, Black JM, Goldberg M, McNichol L, Moore L, Sieggreen M. Revised national pressure ulcer advisory panel pressure injury staging system. Journal of Wound Ostomy and Continence Nursing. 2016;**43**(6):585-597. DOI: 10.1097/won.0000000000000281

[6] Saghaleini SH, Dehghan K, Shadvar K, Sanaie S, Mahmoodpoor A, Ostadi Z. Pressure ulcer and nutrition. Indian Journal of Critical Care Medicine. 2018;**22**(4):283-289. DOI: 10.4103/ijccm.IJCCM_277_17

[7] Chen Y, Cai T, Le P, Zhang L, Chen Y, Wu L, et al. Family caregivers' perceptions and challenges in the care of pressure injuries in daily life: A qualitative study. BMC Geriatrics. 2025;**25**(1):1-14

[8] Siotos C, Bonett AM, Damoulakis G, Becerra AZ, Kokosis G, Hood K, et al. Burden of pressure injuries: Findings from the global burden of disease study. PubMed. 2022;**22**:e19. Available from: https://pubmed.ncbi.nlm.nih.gov/35873067

[9] Borojeny LA, Albatineh AN, Dehkordi AH, Gheshlagh RG. The incidence of pressure ulcers and its associations in different wards of the hospital: A systematic review and meta-analysis. International Journal of Preventive Medicine. 2020;**11**:171. DOI: 10.4103/ijpvm.IJPVM_182_19

[10] Li Z, Lin F, Thalib L, Chaboyer W. Global prevalence and incidence of pressure injuries in hospitalised adult patients: A systematic review and meta-analysis. International Journal of Nursing Studies. 2020;**105**:103546. DOI: 10.1016/j.ijnurstu.2020.103546

[11] Anthony D, Alosaimi D, Shiferaw WS, Korsah K, Safari R. Prevalence of pressure ulcers in Africa: A systematic review and meta-analysis. Journal of Tissue Viability. 2020;**30**(1):137-145. DOI: 10.1016/j.jtv.2020.10.003

[12] Berlowitz DV, VanDeusen Lukas C, Parker V, Niederhauser A, Silver J, Logan C, et al. Preventing pressure ulcers in hospitals: A toolkit for improving quality of care. Rockville, MD: Agency for Healthcare Research and Quality; 2011

[13] Nussbaum SR, Carter MJ, Fife CE, DaVanzo J, Haught R, Nusgart M, et al.

An economic evaluation of the impact, cost, and Medicare policy implications of chronic nonhealing wounds. Value in Health. 2017;**21**(1):27-32. DOI: 10.1016/j.jval.2017.07.007

[14] Padula WV, Delarmente BA. The national cost of hospital-acquired pressure injuries in the United States. International Wound Journal. 2019;**16**(3):634-640. DOI: 10.1111/iwj.13071

[15] Demarré L, Van Lancker A, Van Hecke A, Verhaeghe S, Grypdonck M, Lemey J, et al. The cost of prevention and treatment of pressure ulcers: A systematic review. International Journal of Nursing Studies. 2015;**52**(11):1754-1774. DOI: 10.1016/j.ijnurstu.2015.06.006

[16] Thomas DR, Goode PS, Tarquine PH, Allman RM. Hospital-acquired pressure ulcers and risk of death. Journal of the American Geriatrics Society. 1996;**44**(12):1435-1440. DOI: 10.1111/j.1532-5415.1996.tb04067.x

[17] Zhang S, Wei G, Han L, Zhong W, Lu Z, Niu Z. Global, regional and national burden of decubitus ulcers in 204 countries and territories from 1990 to 2021: A systematic analysis based on the global burden of disease study 2021. Frontiers in Public Health. 2025;**13**:41. DOI: 10.3389/fpubh.2025.1494229

[18] Smith DM, Snow DE, Rees E, Zischkau AM, Hanson JD, Wolcott RD, et al. Evaluation of the bacterial diversity of pressure ulcers using bTEFAP pyrosequencing. BMC Medical Genomics. 2010;**3**(1):41. DOI: 10.1186/1755-8794-3-41

[19] Arnold M, Barbul A. Nutrition and wound healing. Plastic and Reconstructive Surgery. 2006;**117**(SUPPLEMENT):42S-58S. DOI: 10.1097/01.prs.0000225432.17501.6c

[20] Iizaka S, Sanada H, Nakagami G, Sekine R, Koyanagi H, Konya C, et al. Estimation of protein loss from wound fluid in older patients with severe pressure ulcers. Nutrition. 2010;**26**(9):890-895

[21] Gavran L, Pavlović J, Račić M, Ivković N, Bunc KT. Evaluation of biochemical markers effectiveness in elderly malnutrition assessment. Medicinski Glasnik. 2019;**16**(2):351-358

[22] Evans E. Nutritional assessment in chronic wound care. Journal of Wound Ostomy and Continence Nursing. 2005;**32**(5):317-320. DOI: 10.1097/00152192-200509000-00009

[23] Arribas-López E, Zand N, Ojo O, Snowden MJ, Kochhar T. The effect of amino acids on wound healing: A systematic review and meta-analysis on arginine and glutamine. Nutrients. 2021;**13**(8):2498. DOI: 10.3390/nu13082498

[24] Serón-Arbeloa C, Labarta-Monzón L, Puzo-Foncillas J, Mallor-Bonet T, Lafita-López A, Bueno-Vidales N, et al. Malnutrition screening and assessment. Nutrients. 2022;**14**(12):2392. DOI: 10.3390/nu14122392

[25] Stechmiller JK. Understanding the role of nutrition and wound healing. Nutrition in Clinical Practice. 2010;**25**(1):61-68

[26] Australian Wound Management Association. Pan Pacific Clinical Practice Guideline for the Prevention and Management of Pressure Injury. Osborne Park, WA: Cambridge Media; 2012. ISBN Print: 978-0-9807842-5-1 ISBN Online: 978-0-9807842-3-7

[27] Yamamoto T, Fujioka M, Kitamura R, Yakabe A, Kimura H, Katagiri Y, et al.

Evaluation of nutrition in the healing of pressure ulcers: Are the EPUAP nutritional guidelines sufficient to heal wounds? PubMed. 2009;**21**(6):153-157. Available from: https://pubmed.ncbi.nlm.nih.gov/25903438

[28] Demling RH. Nutrition, anabolism, and the wound healing process: An overview. PubMed. 2009;**9**:e9. Available from: https://pubmed.ncbi.nlm.nih.gov/19274069

[29] Trans Tasman Dietetic Wound Care Group. Evidence Based Practice Guidelines for the Nutritional Management of Adults with Pressure Injuries. Australia: Trans Tasman Dietetic Wound Care Group; 2010

[30] Malone-Povolny MJ, Maloney SE, Schoenfisch MH. Nitric oxide therapy for diabetic wound healing. Advanced Healthcare Materials. 2019;**8**(12):1801210. DOI: 10.1002/adhm.201801210

[31] Alexander JW, Supp DM. Role of arginine and omega-3 fatty acids in wound healing and infection. Advances in Wound Care. 2013;**3**(11):682-690. DOI: 10.1089/wound.2013.0469

[32] Zhang X, Chinkes DL, Wolfe RR. The anabolic effect of arginine on proteins in skin wound and muscle is independent of nitric oxide production. Clinical Nutrition. 2008;**27**(4):649-656. DOI: 10.1016/j.clnu.2008.01.006

[33] Irving SY, Berry KG, Morgan S, Seiple SM, Nagle ML, Stetzer M, et al. Nutrition association with skin integrity and pressure injury in critically ill pediatric patients. Nutrition in Clinical Practice. 2023;**38**:S125-S138

[34] Ulutaşdemir N, Ay H, Göçmen A, Uzun S, Kulakaç N. Practices of patient relatives aimed at preventing pressure injuries and their experiences of coping with the burden of care: A qualitative study. Advances in Skin & Wound Care. 2024;**37**(3):1-6. DOI: 10.1097/ASW.0000000000000104

[35] Liu Z, Heffernan C, Tan J. Caregiver burden: A concept analysis. International Journal of Nursing Sciences. 2020;**7**(4):438-445. DOI: 10.1016/j.ijnss.2020.07.012

[36] Kalandari E, Govina O, Tzonichaki I, Adamakidou T, Mantoudi A, Apostolara P, et al. Exploration of the relationship between the burden and family support among family caregivers of older adults with chronic diseases: A cross- sectional study [review of exploration of the relationship between the burden and family support among family caregivers of older adults with chronic diseases: A cross-sectional study]. International Journal of Caring Sciences. 2023;**16**(1):51-61. Available from: https://www.internationaljournalofcaringsciences.org/docs/5.mantzorou.pdf

[37] Toledano-Toledano F, Domínguez-Guedea MT. Psychosocial factors related with caregiver burden among families of children with chronic conditions. BioPsychoSocial Med. 2019;**13**:6. DOI: 10.1186/s13030-019-0147-2

[38] Perez-Escamilla R, Bermudez O, Buccini GS, Kumanyika S, Lutter CK, Monsivais P, et al. Nutrition disparities and the global burden of malnutrition. BMJ. 2018:k2252. DOI: 10.1136/bmj.k2252

[39] Oliveira GAL, Buccini G, Gonçalves VSS, Gubert MB, Toral N. Regular family meals associated with nutritional status, food consumption, and sedentary and eating behaviors of Brazilian schoolchildren and their caregivers. Food. 2024;**13**(23):3975. DOI: 10.3390/foods13233975

[40] Maresova P, Javanmardi E, Barakovic S, Barakovic Husic J, Tomsone S, Krejcar O, et al. Consequences of chronic diseases and other limitations associated with old age–a scoping review. BMC Public Health. 2019;**19**(1):1431

[41] Paul A, Nag P. Global trends of population dynamics oncoming 2050. Population Geography. 2024;**46**:1-26

[42] Rodrigues FR, Tavares DMDS. Resilience in elderly people: Factors associated with sociodemographic and health conditions. Revista Brasileira de Enfermagem. 2021;**74**(Suppl 2):e20200171

[43] Peterson A, Fraix MP, Agrawal DK. Preventing pressure injuries in individuals with impaired mobility: Best practices and future directions. The Journal of Surgical Research. 2025;**8**(3):319

[44] Wright D. Nutrition and hospital mortality, morbidity and health outcomes. In: Strategies to Reduce Hospital Mortality in Lower and Middle Income Countries (LMICs) and Resource-Limited Settings. London, UK: IntechOpen; 2019

[45] Munoz N, Posthauer ME, Cereda E, Schols JM, Haesler E. The role of nutrition for pressure injury prevention and healing: The 2019 international clinical practice guideline recommendations. Advances in Skin and Wound Care. 2020;**33**(3):123-136

[46] Burston A, Miles SJ, Fulbrook P. Patient and carer experience of living with a pressure injury: A meta-synthesis of qualitative studies. Journal of Clinical Nursing. 2023;**32**(13-14):3233-3247

[47] Wright DA. Nutritional care and intervention in spinocerebellar ataxia. In: Ataxia-Practice Essentials and Interventions. London, UK: IntechOpen; 2023

Chapter 4

Crushed by Caregiving: The Growing Burden on Families of Individuals with Substance Use Addiction

Wada Gaolaolwe, Miriam Mmamphamo Moagi,
Keletwaetse Sakwape and Gaotswake Patience Kovane

Abstract

Caregivers frequently encounter significant role strain as they care for family members dealing with substance use and addiction issues. This burden encompasses profound emotional exhaustion and a sense of helplessness as they observe their loved ones grappling with addiction and experiencing withdrawal symptoms. Additionally, family caregivers face financial strain due to the steep costs associated with treatment and rehabilitation. They may also bear the financial repercussions of debts or losses incurred from the actions of the individual with the substance use problem. Despite playing a vital role, these caregivers – often family members – face substantial psychological and social hurdles, particularly in environments where stigma is widespread. As a result, families affected by addiction endure considerable emotional strain, which is further exacerbated by a lack of supportive resources, stigma, and limited access to mental health services.

Keywords: addiction, family, substance use, caregiver, role strain

1. Introduction

There's a growing concern about the challenges faced by caregivers of relatives struggling with substance use or addiction problems [1, 2]. Caregivers, who are usually parents, partners, children, siblings, close relatives, and friends, are deeply impacted by their loved ones' substance misuse. They often experience harm to their financial, mental, emotional, and physical well-being. For the past few decades, the use of illicit drugs has become widespread, affecting nearly every corner of the globe. No society is immune to the devastating effects of substance use. Substance use disorder (SUD) is complex, and its impact extends beyond the individual to families and communities. In the family, a member with SUD deeply affects everyone, with a profound impact on the primary caregiver, who often bears the brunt of the burden.

The effect of substance use can devastate caregivers, strain family relationships, and deplete family financial resources. Family resources cover the high costs of rehabilitation care, which is stressful [3]. Additionally, families face increased stress due to heightened conflicts caused by a member's substance use, which affects the family's stability. Providing support to a family member with an SUD puts a constant strain on caregivers, resulting in stress, anger, depression, and anxiety [4]. The stress is often worsened by feelings of shame and guilt caused by the behavioural problems of the person with substance use problems within the family. Consequently, such families usually face emotional turmoil, unmet needs, weakened bonds, financial difficulties, and even violence. The caregivers constantly endure unanticipated and unbudgeted financial burdens due to emergency medical care, legal problems, and added support needed during addiction treatment. The unforeseen expenses destabilize the families' homeostasis and create long-term financial instability, adding significant stress to the already daunting caregiving responsibilities [3].

2. Walking in their shoes: Experiences of families with a member with SUD

The strain experienced by caregivers as a direct result of the challenging circumstances linked to a close relative's addiction is concerning. Strain refers to the effects that substance use has on a family member's health or well-being. The situation is typically so stressful that it tends to jeopardise their health [5]. Research on families with a member struggling with substance use issues suggests that the substance user is often regarded as the primary cause of family dysfunction and the overall instability of the family. Communication is a vital social skill for effective interpersonal interactions in the family, and substance users may struggle with assertiveness and clear communication. Poor communication from a family member with a substance user can alter the behaviour of the family and impact the entire family system.

Another major concern regarding family caregivers of substance users is the lack of support, resources, and training [6]. Often, especially in families where the substance user is newly diagnosed, caregivers are expected to maintain previous roles and routines, which can threaten homeostasis and shift family dynamics if expectations are not met [7]. Family caregivers who are employed frequently encounter disruptions in their work environment, often missing work, arriving late, or leaving early due to their caregiving responsibilities and the absence of resources such as occupational activities that could engage the substance user and prevent their visits to substance use hotspots [8]. These expectations and demands can lead to conflict within the family or workplace and increase stress levels.

If the person struggling with substance use has a job, it can negatively impact their work performance, as job responsibilities are often ignored, leading to potential dismissal or even resignation. This loss can put a strain on family caregivers [9]. Facing the loss of a member's ability to live independently due to work loss or communication difficulties can cause grief and conflict, leading to a hostile family environment [10]. Although professional services, such as community rehabilitation and external support, might be available, some family caregivers may hesitate to seek them out because of societal stigma [3, 46]. As is well-documented, these psychosocial factors play a significant role in increasing chronic stress [11].

What is also overwhelming to caregivers is their constant worry about their relatives' health, safety, and future, which adds to their concerns about the family's overall functioning [1]. Impaired family functioning and increased family conflicts have substantial indirect effects on the quality of care and support that the caregivers provide to a family member with SUD [12, 13]. The damage caused by a family member's substance use includes arguments, ruined family gatherings, and a higher risk of aggression. Although aggression is not present in all substance users, some do display forms of hostility, such as verbal abuse, irritability, rudeness, criticism, and domineering behaviour.

Equally concerning is the damaging effect on the entire family atmosphere. The family becomes characterised by disagreements about how to handle a relative with substance use problems – for instance, disagreements over whether to give them family valuables like a car or money due to a lack of trust. These differences put a strain on family relations and can wreck marriages. The harm to family relationships stresses caregivers, whose constant concern for the relative is compounded by broader worries about overall family functioning and its future, especially when children are the ones involved in substance use. When one partner struggles with substance use, causing family conflict and possibly separation or divorce, the children are often at high risk of being impacted by the consequences. This can lead to family breakdown, neglect, and various forms of abuse.

Families desperately need resources to help them make sense of their experiences and provide options for coping with their distress [4]. Caregivers consistently report difficulty in finding educational resources to increase their understanding of addiction, its effects, and treatment options. The lack of available resources indicates that healthcare providers may not be adequately informed about how addiction impacts caregivers, ways to support families, or what resources are accessible. A deficiency in support often predicts higher caregiver burden. Interventions targeting substance use and addiction must recognise its effects on families supporting a relative with a SUD. Children are particularly at risk of suffering from the fallout, including family breakdown, parental neglect, and various forms of child abuse. Families seek resources to help them understand their experiences and explore options for managing their heartache [4].

3. Caregiver role strain and substance users' bad behaviour: A bitter pill to swallow

Added to the stress of caregiving is the risk that the family faces because of the life and behaviour of their family member with SUD, which is a bitter pill to swallow. Often, caregivers are exposed to drug dealers because of their family member's connections to drug dealing, which causes the family to live in fear and stress. The caregivers face threats and complaints from others due to public disturbances, criminal or aggressive behaviour of substance users, including theft [3]. These behaviours are often a result of cravings or withdrawal problems and have deleterious social and legal consequences that pose a constant source of fear and stress for families. A corpus of evidence suggests that substance use can either exacerbate or prolong criminal behaviour [14].

Early studies have also found that crime rates tend to be higher during periods marked by substance use. According to O'Donnell [15], narcotic addiction often leads to a rise in criminal activity. The criminal activities include gambling, fighting, and drug dealing [1, 16]. This is because substance use is often tied to compulsive behaviours like gambling, which can lead to financial struggles for families due to debt. In a desperate bid to win, users may gamble large sums daily in an attempt to raise money for drugs, affecting both their personal and family income [16]. Sometimes, users gamble away valuable family possessions to keep playing, causing financial strain, family conflicts, and fights. This can ultimately result in lost family valuables, legal expenses, and a worsening family financial situation.

This puts the family in a stressful situation as they have to grapple with a dire financial impact. The families face detrimental financial consequences that include legal and drug debts created from lending money to feed cravings or even dispossessing other people's valuables to get drugs, despite having to cover high rehabilitation costs [1]. It is evident that, in some cases, to fund their addiction habit, the substance users may resort to theft, adding to the financial strain on caregivers [3]. Ultimately, these illicit activities frequently result in legal repercussions that may compel family members to assume the financial responsibilities associated with court fines, legal expenses, or even incarceration costs [16]. When the substance user is involved in theft or damage to neighbours or community property, the family is compelled to replace the stolen items or borrow funds to compensate the victims.

Some individuals with substance use disorder (ISUD), like those with other psychiatric conditions, may exhibit symptoms that require attention and supervision to maintain stability and avoid substance use. Family members who are the main support for a loved one struggling with addiction to substances often experience a negative impact on their social lives. It's hard for them to take part in social activities or go on holidays because of the unpredictability of their relative's behaviour, especially if they have an addiction. Even at social events or special occasions, they have to be constantly on the lookout for problems and ready to respond quickly. It can be a significant emotional burden, affecting caregivers in a negative way [1].

Although caregivers are affected by the poor quality of their social activities, they are particularly frustrated that they cannot enjoy events they had anticipated enjoying. Caregivers consistently feel unease and a sense of foreboding related to their support role. They are unable to foresee a future where their circumstances improve, as they constantly stress over the next substance use-related incident in their daily family life [1, 3]. They harbour feelings of pessimism about the situation of their family member with addiction problems getting better, leading to a sense of hopelessness, as they see no end to their struggles. Family members' fear and hopelessness are also rooted in their perception that the substance user's situation will worsen with continued use of substances and behaviour that is damaging to both the family and community life [1]. Substance users frequently lose control as a result of the influence of substances and disregard moral boundaries. During episodes of intense cravings, individuals may resort to aggression or threats, even towards close family members, thereby presenting significant safety concerns [3].

4. Stigma of SUD and caregiver role strain

Stigmatisation is a social and psychological process encompassing four fundamental components: labelling, discrimination, stereotyping, and rejection [17, 18]. Erving Goffman, a pioneer in the study of stigma in the 1960s, defined it as a complex social construct that describes how people perceived as having inferior qualities are treated unfairly and negatively [17]. In his work [17], he argued that stigma is an attribute that severely discredits an individual, rendering them tainted and devalued. Stigma has been pinpointed as a key driver of substance dependence and one of the strongest predictors of hesitation to seek treatment, and therefore, a major obstacle to recovery [19, 20].

Stigma has negative effects, including disrupting relationships, harming health, and reducing help-seeking [21, 22, 45]. These effects weaken social ties, increase stress and trauma, and worsen substance use, with the burden being felt by the family due to caregiver role strain. Not only do families struggle with managing addiction behaviour, but they also encounter courtesy stigma related to SUD because of their association with a family member affected by SUD. The experiences of this courtesy stigma, as reported across various studies, reveal multiple manifestations of stigma, including social isolation, self-imposed secrecy, and feelings of shame and guilt [3, 23]. These studies highlight the stigma surrounding SUDs as a major obstacle to seeking support and treatment for individuals with SUDs and their family members. This stigma has been identified as a barrier to accessing vital services, which has had a negative impact on the mental health, decision-making, and overall well-being of family members [24]. Owing to stereotypical depictions of individuals with SUDs, including the stigmatising language employed in policies, families frequently report experiencing social distancing and exclusion, blame manifested through derogatory remarks, and feelings of shame. Consequently, family members often suffer from diminished self-esteem, internalised stigma (self-stigma), and disrupted social relationships with the individual living with SUD as well as with other community members [25].

It's concerning that caregivers face not only the emotional toll of courtesy stigma from the public but also the added stress of structural stigma, which worsens their role as caregivers. Structural discrimination is a type of stigma that occurs through various institutions, and healthcare systems are a primary source of this discrimination for families dealing with SUDs. These families often experience neglect from healthcare providers, who may show a lack of care for both patients and families, creating a negative atmosphere in these settings. As a result, families feel ignored, distanced, and isolated, and are treated without empathy. Structural discrimination also manifests in the lack of public health education about SUD, which makes it harder to combat stigma and obtain the needed support for these families [25, 26].

The cause of stigma towards people with SUD and their families also stems from a lack of understanding of addiction as a neurobiological disease, as it is often viewed as a moral failure on the part of the substance user, as well as a failure on the part of the family to socialise their family member with SUD properly. For centuries, substance use has always been viewed as a moral issue, and substance-related behaviours as a disregard for and violation of societal values [27]. When substance use is viewed as a moral failure, the cause is attributed to an individual's lack of willpower to resist substances due to their inherent moral weakness [27]. However, it is evident that SUD is a brain disease with dysfunction in neurobiological processes as the primary drivers of SUDs, contrary to the moral model that attributes it to personal choice [28]. Pundits of the moral model contend that the view of SUD as a brain disease paints a picture of substance use or misuse as an involuntary compulsion, which is insufficiently supported, while the use of substances is actually a consciously made decision [29]. However, the view of SUDs as moral failure from personal weakness is a cause of concern, as it results in stigma, shame, and blame. The caregivers who suffer public stigma also tend to discriminate against themselves due to internalised prejudice, as they accommodate and perpetuate societal stereotypes towards themselves [30, 31].

This is confirmed by a study conducted by [32], in which caregivers showed a tendency to avoid being identified with a family member who has a mental illness or being seen with them at social events due to shame and embarrassment. The stigma becomes a significant barrier to the support that caregivers must offer to a family member with SUD, resulting in substance use relapses and adding to heightened caregiver role strain [28]. Though the moral model recognizes other influential factors in developing SUD, such as the roles of parents and society in shaping a child's moral character as a risk or protective factor against SUDs.

This perspective, with its emphasis on morality as the genesis of substance use or misuse, generally shifts the public health focus and discussion away from other important risk factors, such as a difficult childhood, growing up in poverty, or experiencing maltreatment [28]. The result is discriminatory behaviours that characterise social stigma, such as labelling, stereotyping, pessimistic prediction, restrictiveness, and prejudice towards others [33, 34, 45]. Consequently, the stigma impedes the realisation of a better quality of life for caregivers and may lead them to exhibit behaviours such as social withdrawal, lack of support for their family member with SUD, and disruption of the family structural framework [31, 35, 45].

5. Substance use relapses and family role strain

The burden experienced by caregivers, attributable to caregiving responsibilities, is exacerbated by relapses into substance use. Individuals who use substances often endure recurrent cycles of relapse, oscillating between phases of active substance consumption and periods of treatment and abstinence, which may extend over several years [36]. This creates a vicious circle. However, many caregivers pin their hopes on the fact that recovery is achievable, though the harsh reality of relapse or the unwillingness of the individual with SUD to seek treatment ultimately diminishes their optimism, resulting in a sense of losing control. This sense of losing control over their loved one's life further intensifies the family's suffering, rendering the caregiving of substance users unbearable for families [3].

The continued relapses stemming from the need to feed the addiction among substance users are pervasive, forming a relentless cycle that creates persistent strain on caregivers, culminating in feelings of being stuck on a dangerous and erratic rollercoaster [37]. Watching a loved one struggle with substance use addiction, often relapsing and alternating between active use and periods of treatment and abstinence, which can last for many years, is heartbreaking for families [36, 38]. Worse, the cost of treatment these families bear during these relapses can be substantial, yet it tends to provide limited long-term benefits. Research suggests that around 65–70% of substance users return to using their primary substances within three months after treatment, and two-thirds relapse within a year [46].

The constant threat of substance use relapse causes intense fatigue for family caregivers, and relapses bring financial strain to cover rehabilitation costs, unwanted deviant behaviour, and social conflicts [3]. Caregivers are always worried about the need for continuous, intensive care before and during treatment, leaving them mentally and physically exhausted. Caregivers in a study by Mubashir [3] reported substantial financial strain caused by high treatment and rehabilitation costs, often facing a dilemma of choosing between essential family needs and covering the cost of care for their loved one, who, after spending so much, trips back into relapse [3]. This financial instability and dilemma heighten the caregivers' emotional stress, especially in the midst of limited resources and support.

6. Strategies for SUD prevention to relieve caregiver role strain

Standing up for someone with SUD requires family caregivers to invest a great deal of effort and time. Family caregivers often attempt to resolve their dilemma by finding a compromise solution to dealing with the behaviour of their family member with SUD, while attempting to provide support and avoid rejecting them [12]. However, informal caregiving puts a significant strain on family members, especially primary caregivers, leading to feelings of being stressed, overwhelmed, and socially isolated.

These individuals often experience a loss of identity and feel 'engulfed' by their caregiving role [6, 39], where their personal identity becomes consumed by their caregiving responsibilities. As their identities shift, they may start to see their caregiving role as a burden [40]. The stress of this situation can take a toll on both their physical and emotional well-being [6]. For the ultimate success of the whole recovery journey, it's essential to care for both the individual with SUD and their caregivers.

Omitting caregivers from the care process creates a gap that undermines the progress of their family member struggling with substance use or addiction. It is worrying that, although addiction clearly has a significant impact on a family's physical and mental health, there is evidence that healthcare providers often overlook the stress caused by the support needed for a relative [4]. Consequently, families may continue to live with unaddressed and unresolved health issues stemming from the challenges of caring for an individual with SUD. Facilitating self-care for families impacted by addiction necessitates acknowledging caregiver distress, which may augment caregivers' capacity to support their loved one's recovery.

Limited understanding of caregiver role strain caused by substance use may overlook the unique needs and challenges faced by both the substance user and their caregivers, which, in turn, hampers the development of targeted preventive strategies for SUD [41]. Thus, the family and individual substance user dynamics have to be taken into account for successful recovery initiatives. As a result, caregivers should be part of the recovery plan for their member undergoing rehabilitation or treatment to ensure its effectiveness and also need to be supported throughout the process. Recovery plans and support initiatives need to take into account the social, cultural, and environmental aspects of the family in question [42].

To ease caregivers' burden and strain, it begins with addressing their main concern: the availability of proper rehabilitation facilities and services for their family member with a SUD [38]. Caregivers may grasp the complexities of substance use and the support they can offer, but if treatment and rehabilitation services are inadequate, they can feel powerless and uncertain about what to do next. Their future as a family becomes clouded by a lingering sense of gloom and uncertainty. Therefore, to ease the caregivers' stress and uncertainties facing them, the family caregivers of individuals experiencing substance use issues require adequate and appropriate social support programmes, such as care for the caregivers.

These programmes foster resilience and ensure caregivers receive counselling and psychoeducational resources to understand SUD as a mental health condition and to manage the stress arising from their caregiving role amid the challenging circumstances of caring for someone with SUD. This approach aims to enhance the caregivers' understanding and consequently enable effective support for their family member's recovery process. In a substance use prevention programme developed by [38], it is advised that families abstain from employing stigmatising language when referring to their family member's substance use. Instead, they are encouraged to actively participate in their care, monitor for signs of relapse, and triggers, and intervene appropriately, with support from family counselling and psychoeducation. Health workers should collaborate to provide support for substance users and their caregivers [38]. A diverse team of therapists and professionals should ensure that, while substance users undergo intensive rehabilitation, their caregivers also receive adequate support and care to reduce caregiving stress and build resilience before the user is discharged from inpatient care. This can equip families to provide ongoing support and give substance users the necessary skills and strategies to cope with stress and resist triggers. To maintain the progress made in inpatient rehabilitation, health workers should continue care through home visits, outreach programs, and virtual check-ups [38, 43].

7. Conclusion

Caregiver role strain in families caring for their members with substance use or addiction problems is a neglected issue, yet it is a substantial cause for concern that requires attention. Family caregivers face inadequate support, stigma, and isolation, with stigma being especially rampant in communities where addiction is viewed as a moral failure [44]. The distress of caregivers is further compounded by legal issues surrounding their family members with SUD, inadequate treatment options, financial hardship, and limited professional services [3]. Psychological distress, including stress and feelings of helplessness, is aggravated by a lack of caregiver-focused education and support systems [12].

Author details

Wada Gaolaolwe[1*], Miriam Mmamphamo Moagi[2], Keletwaetse Sakwape[1] and Gaotswake Patience Kovane[3]

1 School of Nursing, Faculty of Health Sciences, University of Botswana, Gaborone, Botswana

2 Nursing Department, University of Limpopo, Polokwane, South Africa

3 NuMIQ Research Focus Area, Faculty of Health Sciences, North-West University, Mahikeng, South Africa

*Address all correspondence to: gaolaolwew@ub.ac.bw

References

[1] McCann TV, Polacsek M, Lubman DI. Experiences of family members supporting a relative with substance use problems: A qualitative study. Scandinavian Journal of Caring Sciences. 2019;**33**(4):902–911

[2] Orford J. How does the common core to the harm experienced by affected family members vary by relationship, social and cultural factors? Drugs: Education, Prevention and Policy. 2017;**24**(1):9–16

[3] Mubashir AS, Kainaat R, Arafat SY. Challenges faced by caregivers of individuals with substance use disorder in Pakistan: A qualitative study. Health Science Reports. 2025;**8**(7):e71090

[4] Maina G, Ogenchuk M, Phaneuf T, Kwame A. I can't live like that: The experience of caregiver stress of caring for a relative with substance use disorder. Substance abuse treatment. Prevention, and Policy. 2021;**16**(1):11

[5] Sakwape K, Kovane GP, Chukwuere PC, Moagi MM, Machailo R. Exploring the needs of family caregivers of people living with mental illness: A qualitative study in Lobatse, Botswana. BMC Nursing. 2025;**24**(1):183

[6] Kepic M, Randolph A, Hermann-Turner KM. Care for caregivers: Understanding the need for caregiver support. Adultspan Journal. 2019;**18**(1):40–51

[7] Qualls SH. Caregiving families within the long-term services and support system for older adults. American Psychologist. 2016;**71**(4):283

[8] Gordon JR, Pruchno RA, Wilson-Genderson M, Murphy WM, Rose M. Balancing caregiving and work: Role conflict and role strain dynamics. Journal of Family Issues. 2012;**33**(5):662–689

[9] Rawat H, Petzer SL, Gurayah T. Effects of substance use disorder on women's roles and occupational participation. South African Journal of Occupational Therapy. 2021;**51**(1):54–62

[10] Humphrey KM. Counseling Strategies for Loss and Grief. Alexandria, VA: American Counseling Association; 2009

[11] Weinbrecht A, Rieckmann N, Renneberg B. Acceptance and efficacy of interventions for family caregivers of elderly persons with a mental disorder: A meta-analysis. International Psychogeriatrics. 2016;**28**(10):1615–1629

[12] Orford J, Velleman R, Copello A, Templeton L, Ibanga A. The experiences of affected family members: A summary of two decades of qualitative research. Drugs: Education, Prevention and Policy. 2010;**17**(sup1):44–62

[13] Selbekk AS, Sagvaag H. Troubled families and individualised solutions: An institutional discourse analysis of alcohol and drug treatment practices involving affected others. Sociology of Health & Illness. 2016;**38**(7):1058–1073

[14] Hussong AM, Curran PJ, Moffitt TE, Caspi A, Carrig MM. Substance abuse hinders desistance in young adults' antisocial behavior.

Development and Psychopathology. 2004;**16**(4):1029–1046

[15] O'Donnell JA. Narcotic addiction and crime. Social Problems. 1965; **13**:374

[16] Isanzu NH. Effects of alcohol abuse on families' financial stability: A sociological inquiry in Tanzania. Tanzania Journal of Community Development. 2023;**3**(1):113–128

[17] Goffman E. Stigma. London: Penguin; 1963

[18] Pescosolido BA, Martin JK. The stigma complex. Annual Review of Sociology. 2015;**41**(1):87–116

[19] Corrigan P, Schomerus G, Shuman V, Kraus D, Perlick D, Harnish A, Kulesza M, Kane-Willis K, Qin S, Smelson D. Developing a research agenda for understanding the stigma of addictions Part I: Lessons from the mental health stigma literature. The American Journal on Addictions. 2017;**26**(1):59–66

[20] Hammarlund R, Crapanzano KA, Luce L, Mulligan L, Ward KM. Review of the effects of self-stigma and perceived social stigma on the treatment-seeking decisions of individuals with drug-and alcohol-use disorders. Substance Abuse and Rehabilitation. 2018;**9**:115–136

[21] Rüsch N, Angermeyer MC, Corrigan PW. Mental illness stigma: Concepts, consequences, and initiatives to reduce stigma. European Psychiatry. 2005;**20**(8):529–539

[22] Sickel AE, Seacat JD, Nabors NA. Mental health stigma update: A review of consequences. Advances in Mental Health. 2014;**12**(3):202–215

[23] Monari EN, Booth R, Forchuk C, Csiernik R. Experience of family members of relatives with substance use disorders: An integrative literature review. Creative Nursing. 2024;**30**(3):232–244

[24] Clement S, Schauman O, Graham T, Maggioni F, Evans-Lacko S, Bezborodovs N, Morgan C, Rüsch N, Brown JS, Thornicroft G. What is the impact of mental health-related stigma on help-seeking? A systematic review of quantitative and qualitative studies. Psychological Medicine. 2015;**45**(1): 11–27

[25] Bhatia U, Gandhi Y. Stigma as a barrier to care as experienced by affected family members. In: Bischof G, et al, editors. Families Affected by Addiction, Sustainable Development Goals Series: A Handbook Cham Springer Nature Switzerland. 2025. p. 155–165

[26] Dobener LM, Fahrer J, Purtscheller D, Bauer A, Paul JL, Christiansen H. How do children of parents with mental illness experience stigma? A systematic mixed studies review. Frontiers in Psychiatry. 2022;**13**:813519

[27] Frank LE, Nagel SK. Addiction and moralization: The role of the underlying model of addiction. Neuroethics. 2017;**10**(1):129–139

[28] Rampa S, Molebatsi K, January J. Aetiology and early developmental influences on substance use disorders. In: Mhaka-Mutepfa M, editor. Substance Use and Misuse in sub-Saharan Africa: Trends, Intervention, and Policy. Cham: Springer International Publishing; 2022. p. 17–30

[29] Pickard H. What we're not talking about when we talk about addiction. Hastings Center Report. 2020;**50**(4): 37–46

[30] Corrigan PW. Lessons learned from unintended consequences about erasing the stigma of mental illness. World Psychiatry. 2016;**15**(1):67–73

[31] Kamaradova D, Latalova C, Prasko J, Kubinik R, Vrbova K, Mainerova B, . . . Tichackova A. Connection between self-stigma, adherence to treatment, and continuation of medication. PMC Journal. 2016;**10**(1):1289–1298

[32] Girma E, Möller-leimkühler AM, Dehning S, Mueller N, Tesfaye M, Froeschl G. Self-stigma among care-givers of people with mental illness: Toward caregiver empowerment. Journal of Multidisciplinary Healthcare. 2014;**7** (1):37–43

[33] Becker TD, Ho-Foster AR, Poku OB, Marobela S, Mehta H, Cao DTX, Yang LH. "It's when the trees blossom": explanatory beliefs, stigma, and mental illness in the context of HIV in Botswana. SAGE Journals. 2019;**29** (11):1566–1580

[34] Poreddi V, Blrudu R, Math SB. Mental health literacy among caregivers of persons with mental illness. Journal of Neurosciences in Rural Practice. 2015;**6**(3):355–360

[35] Milačić-Vidojević I, Gligorović M, Dragojević N. Tendency towards stigmatization of families of a person with autistic spectrum disorders. International Journal of Social Psychiatry. 2014;**60** (1):63–70

[36] Strang J, Volkow ND, Degenhardt L, Hickman M, Johnson K, Koob GF, Marshall BD, Tyndall M, Walsh SL. Opioid use disorder. Nature Reviews Disease Primers. 2020;**6**(1): 1–28

[37] Weimand BM, Birkeland B, Ruud T, Høie MM. "It's like being stuck on an unsafe and unpredictable rollercoaster": Experiencing substance use problems in a partner. Nordic Studies on Alcohol and Drugs. 2020;**37** (3):227–242

[38] Gaolaolwe W, Moagi MM, Kovane GP, Sehularo L. Exploration of effective substance use relapse prevention programmes for the youth: An integrative literature review. Journal of Psychiatric and Mental Health Nursing. 2025;**32**(3):661–679

[39] Eifert EK, Adams R, Dudley W, Perko M. Family caregiver identity: A literature review. American Journal of Health Education. 2015;**46**(6):357–367

[40] Grunfeld E, Coyle D, Whelan T, Clinch J, Reyno L, Earle CC, Willan A, Viola R, Coristine M, Janz T, Glossop R. Family caregiver burden: Results of a longitudinal study of breast cancer patients and their principal caregivers. Canadian Medical Association Journal. 2004;**170**(12):1795–1801

[41] Moe FD, Moltu C, McKay JR, Nesvåg S, Bjornestad J. Is the relapse concept in studies of substance use disorders a 'one size fits all' concept? A systematic review of relapse operationalisations. Drug and Alcohol Review. 2022;**41**(4):743–758

[42] Maikano KL, Mogomotsi RP, Diraditsile K, Jeremiah RP. Prevention and intervention for substance Use/ Misuse. In: Mhaka-Mutepfa M, editor. Substance Use andMisuse in sub-Saharan Africa. Trends, Intervention

and Policy. Cham: Palgrave Macmillan; 2021. p. 161–175

[43] WHO-UNODC. International standards for the treatment of drug use disorders: Revised edition incorporating results of field-testing. 2020. Available from: https://www.unodc.org [Accessed: 2025-September-21]

[44] Ayers C, Manthey M, Choflet A. Substance use disorder: From moral failure to disease management. In: Davidson JE, Richardson M, editors. Workplace Wellness: From Resiliency to SuicidePrevention and Grief Management: A Practical Guide to Supporting Healthcare Professionals. Cham: Springer International Publishing; 2023. p. 309–321

[45] Gaolaolwe W, Manyedi E, Serapelwane M. Family members' experiences of courtesy stigma associated with mental illness. Health SA Gesondheid. 2023;**28**(1).

[46] Gonzales-Castaneda R, McKay JR, Steinberg J, Winters KC, Yu CH, Valdovinos IC, Casillas JM, McCarthy KC. Testing mediational processes of substance use relapse among youth who participated in a mobile texting aftercare project. Substance Abuse. 2022;**43**(1):1–2

Chapter 5

Perspective Chapter: Cultural Patterns and Outcomes of Umbilical Cord Care in Africa – Implications for Neonatal Health and Long-Term Development

Elaunire Monica Agianipe, Ndep Antor Odu, Akpan Margaret Inemiesit, Undie Emmanuel Ugbong and Efut Joseph Ajah

Abstract

Cultural beliefs and practices regarding childbirth and early child care have a strong effect on neonatal health outcomes in Africa, particularly with umbilical cord care. The chapter critically examines the effectiveness of different African practices for managing the umbilical cord of neonates. Drawing upon a comprehensive review of ethnographic research, clinical health assessments, and empirical studies, the chapter discusses how specific methods that utilize herbs, ashes, cow dung, or other non-sterile substances have been associated with increased risks of neonatal infection, sepsis, and mortality. It also highlights the positive impact of evidence-based interventions like chlorhexidine gel, while paying attention to cultural practices that have facilitated both community acceptance and improved health outcomes. The chapter underscores the importance of caring for newborns by respecting other community members' beliefs, as we advance neonatal safety and promote optimal growth and development. Plans to harmonize traditional beliefs with contemporary medical practices should involve sharing expertise and coordinating efforts among researchers, community workers, and policymakers.

Keywords: cultural patterns, outcomes, umbilical cord, cord care, neonatal health

1. Introduction

Newborn survival and early healthy growth rely on appropriate care of the umbilical cord, especially in low- and middle-income countries (LMICs), where the hygienic conditions of delivery and the postnatal care settings are often poor. The umbilical stump, when poorly handled – as is the case when it is not managed in a sterile environment – becomes a major point of invasion by microbes and an open gateway to pathogens. This pathway predisposes the neonate to serious infections like neonatal sepsis and omphalitis (infection of the umbilical stump), which are major complications and leading causes of neonatal mortality that can otherwise be prevented [1].

Umbilical cord care is also a cornerstone of newborn survival and healthy early growth, particularly in LMICs, where the level of clean delivery and good postnatal care settings is often compromised. The umbilical stump, unless treated in a sterile environment, poses a major site of invasion by microbes since it acts as an open door to pathogens. This route predisposes the neonate to severe infections like omphalitis (infection of the umbilical stump) and neonatal sepsis, which are major factors resulting in avoidable deaths in neonates [1].

Neonatal infections (particularly omphalitis and neonatal sepsis) contribute to about one-third of all neonatal deaths in Sub-Saharan Africa; thus, cord cleaning as well as evidence-based cord care is a priority of public health [2, 3]. Nonetheless, most African communities still carry out these practices in a traditional way that typically includes the use of substances such as shea butter, cow manure, ash, or herbs, some of which can be harmful in terms of introducing harmful pathogens [4]. These cultural traditions usually go against what is suggested biomedically, and so they continue to contribute to high neonatal infections and mortality rates.

The World Health Organization (WHO) has included actual directions that suggest how dry cord care, the technique of leaving the stump free of any covering and exposed to air, is the safest technique provided clean delivery conditions are met. In regions where there is poor hygiene and a high risk of infection, the WHO recommends the use of a 7.1% concentration of chlorhexidine digluconate (which is equivalent to 4% chlorhexidine) for daily cord cleaning during the first week of life [5]. Clinical evidence has shown that the application of chlorhexidine to the cord may significantly reduce infections and mortality in neonates [6]. Nevertheless, there is still insufficient implementation of this life-saving intervention, especially in rural and underserved areas of Africa, where neonatal care practices remain influenced by traditional customs and spiritual beliefs [4, 7].

In this chapter, the author examines the issue of umbilical cord care as part of African cultures entirely. It questions tradition-specific local practices and related health consequences, as well as the cultural explanations thereof. In addition, it argues for the use of community interventions that have effectively harmonized the divide between traditional and evidence-based care, as well as the usefulness of culturally sensitive health messages in enhancing outcomes toward neonatal care. Finally, the chapter draws attention to the broader policy ramifications, research and agenda setting, and long-term development policy.

2. Overview of cultural practices across African Regions

In the East Mamprusi District of Ghana, a mixture of shea butter, salt, and fowl feces is used to hasten cord separation, which the caregivers infer is necessary to carry out timely naming ceremonies, ensure the protection of the child by its ancestors, and strengthen the newborn [3]. In Nigeria, a paste made of oily materials such as shea oil or palm oil is used, and the stump of the cord is bound with hair or threads before the cord is allowed to dry to block the influences of evil and to ensure the cord separates quickly [4].

In Zambia and Tanzania, substances such as charcoal, ash, herbal pastes, and cow dung are used depending on whether the cord is determined to be too dry or is detaching too slowly; some believe that the cord length influences future fertility [5, 6]. Pig oil or clay powders are added to the cord applications of the VhaVenda and Vatsonga people of South Africa, and this is said to help heal and prevent spiritual harm to the newborn [7].

The umbilical cord is generally seen as the portal through which malignant spirits or disease are able to enter; premature separation or careless disposal is believed to hinder fertility or attract curses [3, 6]. Rapid separation – usually in a few days or a week – is of great value and regarded as a mark of health and spiritual wholesomeness, and therefore caregivers administer wetting or softening agents.

3. Health outcomes associated with traditional cord care methods

3.1 Epidemiological evidence

Various studies have established the fact that the use of nonsterile chemicals on the stump of the umbilical cord actually raises the chances of infection among neonates. It was observed through a systematic review of 17 empirical studies in sub-Saharan Africa that, out of a total of 5,725 caregivers included, neonates who had been in contact with unsafe cord care practices were 13 times more at risk of developing sepsis compared to those following medically recommended care [1]. Such unsanitary at-home practices consisted of using ash, fowl feces, cow dung, and herbal pastes, which usually contain pathogenic bacteria or spores.

The review also showed that about 75% of neonates whose caretakers employed traditional substances of a non-clinical nature recorded clinical signs of infection during the first week of life. Fever, abdominal redness or swelling, pus production, and in severe cases, convulsions or poor feeding were some of the signs. The inflammatory process of the cord and the growth of bacteria in an environment characterized by the pathology of omphalitis are most often the preconditions of neonatal sepsis, which is characterized by systemic inflammation that can be lethal when left unaddressed for a short period of time [1].

This observation gives the highest weightage to the importance of a re-assessment of the cultural aspects and the expansion of public health education to focus on safe, sterile cord practices as an irreplaceable component of neonatal survival interventions.

3.2 Risk of mortality in Northern Nigeria

The ramifications of traditional practices of cord care are particularly severe in places such as Sokoto and Bauchi States in northern Nigeria, where over 80% of births take place outside formal health facilities. In this case, challenges in the availability of a sterile delivery environment and skilled providers increase the vulnerability of neonates. Research carried out in such regions indicated that unsafe cord care was highly proportional to the rate of neonatal mortality [4]. The contamination of the umbilical cord stump in these environments becomes a source of active systemic infection, which is one of the major causes of the high neonatal mortality rate in Nigeria, a country that continues to have one of the highest neonatal mortality rates in the world.

The use of low-cost antiseptic interventions, such as chlorhexidine digluconate gel (7.1%, translating to 4% chlorhexidine), was found to be effective, and it considerably enhanced the outcomes of newborns in the set-L phase. The application of chlorhexidine was linked to a remarkable reduction in omphalitis and sepsis when it was made accessible through community distribution systems, such as neighborhood women's groups and trained birth attendants available in their communities [4]. This demonstrates the capability of community-based models of healthcare delivery to be very useful in settings where formal clinical provisions are unavailable or underutilized.

3.3 Cord care in Eastern Uganda

A prospective cohort study in the east of Uganda supports further life-saving capacity of chlorhexidine. In this work, mothers whose postnatal care regimen included chlorhexidine gel reported a significant decrease in the rates of omphalitis to only 3%, whereas control groups experienced rates of omphalitis that reached up to 52% without the antiseptic treatment to prevent this condition [8]. The study population involved both in-facility and home births, which were informative in regard to contextual risks.

Notably, the survey identified that the neonates born at home were twice as likely to acquire infections of the umbilical cords in comparison to those born in healthcare facilities [8]. This observation represents the twofold impact of the delivery setting and delivery practices on the development of neonatal health. With unskilled birth attendants or family members present during home deliveries, there was a lack of necessary infection prevention practices, so even simple antiseptic methods, such as the use of chlorhexidine, became vital.

3.4 Effectiveness of chlorhexidine

High-quality meta-analyses, including several randomized controlled trials in low-income countries across the world, provide strong evidence regarding the analgesic treatment of chlorhexidine cord care [9, 10]. When 4% chlorhexidine was applied to the umbilical stump, a relative decrease in omphalitis incidence by 35% and a 21% reduction in neonatal deaths were recorded compared to dry cord management or conventional procedures [11]. The findings endorse the WHO recommendations and highlight the potential of chlorhexidine as an inexpensive and scalable intervention for improving newborn survival in resource-limited settings.

Nonetheless, one of the trade-offs noted is a slower process of separation of the umbilical cord, estimated to occur 2.7 days later [12, 13]. Although this delay has been mentioned as one of the caregiver concerns, as they would traditionally interpret swift cord detachment as a sign of a healthy child, the medical opinion has been that there is no harm in this delay, and the advantages of preventing infections far outweigh this slight difference in physiological timing [14].

4. Successful community-based interventions and innovations

4.1 Chlorhexidine roll-out initiatives

Integrated healthcare and supply chain channels have been one of the most successful community-based measures in mitigating umbilical cord infections, mostly through systematically rolling out chlorhexidine. A number of USAID (United States Agency for International Development)-covered projects in Nigeria, Nepal, and Bangladesh have been the first to adopt this strategy, integrating chlorhexidine into national essential drug lists and local supply chains, making availability regular even at the additional birth attendants (traditional birth attendants (TBAs)), community health extension workers (CHEWs), and faith-based organizations by leveraging the influence they have in their localities. The success of the initiative was closely related to local trust, particularly when presented by local and trusted leaders like TBAs, elders, and royal rulers when the chlorhexidine packs were introduced. Of note, the intervention was legitimized by traditional leaders, which not only supported its deployment but also indicated that it was acceptable to the rest of the community [10].

The availability of the products, the cultural mediators, and the local trainings brought about adoption both in rural and peri-urban regions. The pilot sites (Sokoto, Bauchi, and Cross River States) evaluation revealed that maternal acceptance has already grown significantly, particularly when the gel is introduced as a supplementary tool, and not a substitute for the current care practices.

4.2 Communication for behavior change

Implementing behavior change communication (BCC) strategies that fit the local cultural and social contexts of target populations has also been found to be another important ingredient of successful intervention. Both in Zambia and Nigeria, participatory, dialog-based interventions were more sustainable as opposed to one-way health messaging [3, 5].

An example is the Mother-to-Mother support groups that provided a safe space where women could share their experiences and exchange ideas at the community level [8].

The country of Nigeria was strategic in the distribution model that has integrated thoughtful care of the cords together with learning experiences of both trained peers and elder mothers. Open discussion of the safe practices involving TBAs served to demystify biomedical products such as chlorhexidine, thus leaving a breathing space between the modern health advocates and the traditional custodians.

Moreover, the BCC campaigns made use of local languages, visual narration, folk songs, and local theatrics, which together connected more with the listeners of different literacy levels. Such channels, which are culturally embedded, not only minimized resistance but also went on to strengthen appropriate behaviors, particularly in first-time mothers and caregivers who are molded by elder female relatives.

4.3 Hybrid models of cord care

Understanding the difficulty of getting rid of established traditions, various programs took hybrid forms, incorporating some aspects of the antiseptic care of cords along with the cultural rituals. Examples can be found in some areas in the north of Nigeria and western Kenya, where families had the choice to apply chlorhexidine first before using a thin layer of a familiar, culturally acceptable component, such as shea butter or herbal powder, after a specified time [5, 8].

Despite the WHO dry cord care regulation, these were agreed-upon compromises that created confidence and progressive behavior change. Such a trade-off was a so-called harm-reduction strategy in public health terms, according to which the implementation of antiseptic treatment was prioritized, albeit with the toleration of non-toxic rituals in the form of secondary, non-conflicting practices.

Such models also facilitated a conversational co-creation pathway within which community norms and biomedical evidence did not have to be rejected wholesale in order to allow traditional beliefs to exist. Cultural humility exhibited by health workers also resulted in positive compliance levels and reduced cases of omphalitis and neonatal deaths, thereby registering high levels of compliance using the hybrid approach [8].

5. Cultural competence and public health messaging

5.1 Ethnographic insights

The concept of the symbolism of the umbilical cord has its regional perception, which is necessary to comprehend in order to develop effective interventions. Anthropology has revealed that, to most African communities, the umbilical cord is more than a biological tissue; it signifies connection with ancestors as well as spiritual and posterity-fertility [4].

According to the beliefs of some human tribes, the cord associates the baby with ancestry, serves as a form of protection, or helps to predict future prosperity. Such symbolic use influences the substances used, the location of the burial of the cord, and the people permitted to touch it.

It is, therefore, advisable through ethnographic research that the contextual presentation of health messages ought not to confront these viewpoints; instead, it should embrace them. As an example, chlorhexidine may be referred to as a "blessing oil" or a "protective gel," wording that does not affect local ontologies but reinforces them. This critical strategy should be included to achieve culturally appropriate communication as well as reduce resistance.

5.2 The role of TBAs

The TBAs are also highly influential social capital and can be the first people to consult when it comes to childbirth in rural or underserved communities. It is thus not impractical to consider that their sustained participation is strategic. The trend in programs that viewed TBAs more as partners and not as roadblocks significantly improved attitudes toward the acceptance and correct usage of antiseptics such as chlorhexidine [8].

The training interventions aimed at TBAs, focusing on preventing infection, hand hygiene, and the stepwise use of chlorhexidine, were very effective. The TBAs became highly effective agents of change when their status was elevated by respecting them as holders of knowledge and providing them with tools that enhanced their standing. The fact that they endorsed new practices added credibility to them in community conversations, especially among older women and pregnant women.

Instead of removing conventional roles, such strategies involved them in the existing crowd in a manner that contributes to a mutualistic approach to maternal and neonatal care.

5.3 Locally tailored messaging tools

The health information in standard leaflet form or posters with a lot of writing can easily be unsuccessful in delivery where the literacy level is low in the community. New approaches such as community radio programs, pictorial pamphlets, radio plays that are dramatized and sent via mobile phone in the form of SMS reminders have been found to be effective beyond words in behavior change campaigns.

The use of radio plays with sympathetic characters (e.g., Mama Nkechi or Uncle Bala), which dramatized stories of birth where proper health messages were conveyed, was widely listened to in social gatherings in Nigeria. Local theater companies performed live in certain areas, showing how dangerous it is to handle the umbilical cord in an unsafe manner, to generate discussion and encourage reflection on the issue.

Visual aids were also used: examples of posters with step-by-step graphic instructions were posted to ensure that nonliterate mothers could easily carry out safe cord care. Text messages were used as reminders of the postnatal schedules in urban and peri-urban settings, where feasible, due to mobile penetration.

These multi-modal, locally relevant communication strategies significantly improved message retention. These locally relevant communication strategies, through multi-modal communication effectiveness, contributed greatly to message retention and behavior adoption behavior, particularly among first-time mothers and caregivers of low socioeconomic status.

6. Implications for policy, research, and long-term development

6.1 Recommendations to policy

Ministries of Health must incorporate chlorhexidine (or dry care, where feasible) into the national newborn care policy, facilitate and promote local production, and train local actors at the community level to implement culturally adapted messaging interventions.

6.2 Future research

It requires longitudinal studies to assess the impact of preventing infections in newborns by using safe cord care practices, as compared to improved cognitive and physical development. The effectiveness of culturally focused interventions should be tested in different regions of Africa through comparative research.

6.3 Sweeping development impact

Neonatal sepsis reduces the chances of survival, leads to long-term impairments, affects school readiness, and ultimately impacts maternal well-being and community resilience [11] (**Table 1**).

6.3.1 Integrating cultural and health perspectives in cord care in African settings

In most African societies, childbirth is not only a biological process but also a process that is highly spiritual and cultural. With respect to traditional beliefs, rituals, and practices during conception, pregnancy, childbirth, and the post-childbirth period, the mother and the newborn are treated in a specific way. A major element of this continuum is the care of the umbilical cord, which can have symbolic and protective implications within various societies.

Although these traditions serve as recognitions and identifications of the community and motherly attributes, they at times conflict with the biomedical methods, particularly when they pose health threats to the newborn child. Nonetheless, the combination of cultural knowledge and scientific knowledge provides an attractive method of achieving respectful, effective, and culturally competent healthcare.

6.3.2 Cultural perspectives on cord care

In Africa, the umbilical cord is not just a physical bond between a mother and her child, but it is also regarded as a spiritual and social bond. There is cultural diversity involving cord beliefs: The cord is believed to be a means through which spirits or blessings of the ancestors can come to them; therefore, herbal or metaphorical treatments of protection are necessary in most communities in the Nigerian world.

The rate at which the cord falls is considered to be influenced by a certain supernatural interference, whereby a slow fall is seen as a reflection of spiritual struggle or poor health. Beliefs about protecting, drying, or purifying the cord are achieved using substances such as clay, charcoal, palm oil, and breast milk to seal the skin. Depending on the child's status within the cosmic and social order, the cord stump may be ceremonially buried, cast into rivers, or saved to be used ritually. Such traditions are not just forms of folklore but provide a sense of local control, maternal duty, and continuity with ancestral knowledge.

6.3.3 Risk and health perspective

The stump of the umbilical cord serves as a possible source of infection, medically speaking, in neonates whose immune systems are not yet mature. Primarily, neonatal sepsis is the leading cause of death during the first month of life in many countries, and unsafe cord care is one of the major risk factors in resource-poor contexts. Clean cord care, which may be done either as dry care (no contact or attention is given to the stump, and it is kept dry) or by the use of antiseptics like chlorhexidine, especially in situations of high mortality, is encouraged by biomedical guidelines.

Nevertheless, the use of dangerous foodstuffs, lack of hygiene, and the view that some of the delays in cord detachment are to be treated result in the adoption of practices that lead to the following:

Substance used	Cultural rationale	Method of application	Associated health risks	Documented locations
Shea butter	Believed to soften the cord, ease detachment, and protect the child spiritually.	Applied directly to cord stump.	May promote bacterial growth in unsterile conditions; risk of sepsis.	Northern Nigeria, Ghana [3, 5]
Fowl feces	Applied to "dry" the cord quickly and prevent bad spirits.	Smeared on the stump or mixed with oil.	High bacterial load; omphalitis, tetanus, neonatal sepsis.	Nigeria [3]
Petroleum jelly	Keeps the cord moist and prevents cracking; believed to protect future fertility.	Coated on stump post-delivery	Non-sterile containers pose a contamination risk; prolong stump detachment.	Zambia, Malawi, Southern Africa [5, 6]
Charcoal dust	Used to "burn out evil" and hasten cord separation.	Rubbed or sprinkled onto the cord.	Contains carbon particles and impurities; risk of local infection.	Zambia, Tanzania [5]
Cow dung	Believed to pass on strength and vitality from cattle to child.	Packed around or spread over a cord.	Extremely high risk of Clostridium tetani infection; leads to neonatal tetanus.	Pastoral communities in East Africa [5, 6]
Burnt pumpkin stem	Traditionally considered a disinfectant and a symbol of fertility.	Ground to powder and dusted on the cord stump.	May contain spores; insufficient antimicrobial effect; risk of sepsis.	Central Uganda, parts of Tanzania [4, 5]
Salty water or brine	Used to "wash away evil blood" or hasten drying.	Applied with a cloth or cotton wool.	Risk of tissue irritation and possible contamination from unclean water.	Southeastern Nigeria, Cameroon [3, 8]
Ash (wood or herbal)	Purifies the cord, protects from spiritual harm.	Sprinkled over stumps or used with other mixtures.	May introduce fungi or spores; poor hygiene poses risks.	Benin, rural Ghana [5]

Substance used	Cultural rationale	Method of application	Associated health risks	Documented locations
Palm oil	Believed to have soothing, healing, and protective powers; sometimes seen as a blessing or a fertility enhancer.	Applied directly to the cord stump with cotton wool or fingers, often daily, to soften it or help the stump fall off quickly.	Palm oil is not sterile and can readily be contaminated during extraction, handling, and/or storage. It holds moisture, which creates a hot and wet environment, thereby acting as an incubator that allows bacteria to grow. Applying palm oil on the cord stump also contributes to the threat of umbilical cord infection (omphalitis), particularly in cases of poor hygienic conditions. Delayed cord separation may occur due to the naturally retarded drying caused by the presence of moisture from the oil, making infection a likely outcome.	Nigeria [3]
Toothpaste	Considered to "dry up" the stump quickly and keep it clean due to its strong scent and menthol content.	Smeared over the cord stump once or multiple times a day, it is believed to accelerate drying and separation.	Fluoride, abrasives, menthol, and preservatives in toothpaste can burn and irritate newly surfaced baby skin. These compounds can cause skin irritation, dermal burns, or necrosis at the stump site. Toothpaste creates a thick layer that stops air flow, hindering the natural drying process along with cord separation. When the tissue becomes damaged or dead, it becomes more prone to bacterial colonization, leading to infections or sepsis.	Nigeria [3]

Substance used	Cultural rationale	Method of application	Associated health risks	Documented locations
Clay mixed with saliva	Thought to cool, protect, or spiritually cleanse the stump; saliva may be added as part of traditional rituals.	Clay is mixed with human saliva and molded into a paste, which is applied to the cord stump to "draw out bad blood" or connect the child to ancestral earth elements.	Environmental pathogenic bacteria are usually present in clay; among them is Clostridium tetani, which causes neonatal tetanus. There are oral bacteria and viruses that the saliva of a human carries, including Streptococcus, herpes simplex virus, or even hepatitis in specific cases. By rubbing this concoction on the stump, one can cause severe infections such as omphalitis, tetanus, and sepsis. Application and preparation are usually very unhygienic, raising microbial heavy loads and the risk of exposure to pathogens.	Nigeria [3]
Breastmilk	Breast milk is regarded as natural, sacred, and healing in most African and traditional demographics. It is assumed to be spiritually pure and medicinal and is directly transmitted from the mother to the child. The reason behind this belief is the fact that, because breast milk nourishes the baby internally, it can also treat the baby on the outside when it is applied to wounds like the umbilical cord stump. There is also a belief in some cultures that placing breast milk onto the cord brings blessings, prevents evil spirits, and causes the stump to dry and detach easily.	The breastfeeding mother, or the mother who can express her milk, utilizes a couple of drops of her breast milk and rubs it on her fingertips or a slightly wet cloth over the cord stump. This can be performed once or twice a day, especially following the cleaning up or a bath of the newborn. Plainly, in some instances, the application continues until the stump breaks off and, after that, in case it shows any indication of drying or surfacing with scabs.	The fact is that breast milk is not sterile because it can harbor the mother's bacteria, even though it possesses antibodies and antimicrobial agents. Escherichia coli and Staphylococcus aureus may be introduced through expression and the use of unwashed hands. When the cord stump is left with the sugar and fat in breast milk, they serve as a culture medium for bacteria. Breast milk contains moisture, which increases drying time and delays cord separation, hence putting the infant at a risk of infection.	Zambia, Malawi, Nigeria, Southern Africa [5, 6]

Table 1.
Traditional cord substances, cultural rationales, and health risks.

Incrementally increases the risk of tetanus, omphalitis, and systemic infections.

Slow the healing and encourage bacterial growth due to retained moisture agents (such as petroleum jelly or palm oil).

Vague symptoms of an infection, resulting in slow medical-seeking behavior.

Nevertheless, the tendency to condemn cultural practices entirely drives distrust in the mainstream health system further away, which forces caregivers to clinics and skilled care.

6.3.4 Relevance of cultural beliefs to the health system

Cultural assumptions about how to deal with the cords are not necessarily dangerous; it is the specific way it is done and the medical validation that is missing that makes some practices unsafe. Cultural traditions offer an opportunity to design better and stronger health interventions by the community, as their value and influence can be recognized.

Cultural practices can enhance maternal health-seeking behavior when engaged respectfully. For example:

Peer education and care can also be used in the communal approach to traditional care.

Rituals and signs can be maintained, with the dangerous substances being replaced by safe ones.

Holding moral authority, elders and TBAs can be utilized as change agents when included in health education.

Consequently, modern practice is not relevant in the rejection of tradition but in accommodating the positive features of the tradition and making it a part and parcel of the newer model.

6.3.5 Adapting traditional practices for population health

Explain the biomedical reasons for infection control using local traditions based on stories and symbolism. Assuming that the view of the cord is sacred, the message shall be structured in the following way: The cord is sacred, and hence it should be the cleanest and safest; therefore, it is essential to take care of it.

Instead of talking about caregivers doing nothing, the health systems can initiate the use of acceptable alternatives (e.g., chlorhexidine gel) as a modern anointing oil or a holy solution recommended by both health professionals and ancestors.

To make interventions work, TBAs, grandmothers, and traditional healers should take part in designing and delivering interventions and gain confidence and compliance with a program. The experience they have to offer can be used to chart which beliefs can be changed or those that require change.

Cultural sensitivity can be mainstreamed within national policies to ensure that training manuals and maternal health campaigns adopt the use of local languages, metaphors, and practices.

Certain folk medicines (e.g., shea butter or herbal ash) can contain actual antiseptics. Funding ethnobotanical research would make these substances safe to use and allow them to be used on a larger scale to treat the population, turning local knowledge into an acceptable solution to a large-scale problem: local health.

It is possible to create culturally acceptable and relatable health systems containing sterile equipment, chlorhexidine, and photos accompanied by guides based on corresponding cultural signs and images.

7. Recommendations

Based on the findings and the discussions provided in this chapter, it is quite clear that the culture of umbilical cord care has a strong influence on the practice of cord care in Africa due to the traditional belief system, the community system of knowledge, and the inter-generational tradition of care giving. Although certain practices are consistent with or correlate with biomedical guidelines, some of them are seriously life-threatening to neonates and might lead to avoidable morbidity and death.

Therefore, the following recommendations are made to guide policy, research, and practice:

1. When intervening health-wise, one should not strive to eliminate the cultural beliefs but instead complement them. Midwives, community health workers, and nurses are encouraged to be trained in cultural sensitivity to enable them to adopt respectful and collaborative means of approaching the traditional caregivers.

2. Include the TBAs, grandmothers, and spiritual leaders in the development and sharing of the cord care guidelines. They will create a sense of ownership, minimize resistance to change, and make safer options easier to adopt, particularly on a mass scale.

3. The NGOs and governments should advertise and distribute cord-care products – say, chlorhexidine gel – in culturally appealing forms (as protective blessings or as ancestral oils). Messages and packaging need to be presented in the local language and imagery, as well as proverbs, to promote acceptance.

4. The importance of community caregivers to the neonatal health phenomenon should be positively emphasized by national and regional policies. These policies should provide guidelines on training, supervision, and collaboration with traditional caregivers, based on WHO recommendations regarding the care of newborns.

5. Although unsafe practices ought to be prevented, culturally safe and effective practices should be maintained and recorded. This will not only safeguard native knowledge but also will help lead to culture-based health education programs.

8. Conclusion

Umbilical cord care in Africa is influenced by diverse cultural traditions that carry both risks and benefits. While some traditional practices pose threats to neonatal health, others represent valuable knowledge that can be harmonized with biomedical standards. A culturally sensitive, community-based approach integrating traditional birth attendants, evidence-based practices, and respectful public health messaging holds great promise for improving neonatal outcomes across the continent.

Interventions must continue to honor cultural beliefs while prioritizing the health and development of African children. Policymakers, researchers, and practitioners must collaborate with communities to develop sustainable, context-specific strategies that reduce neonatal mortality and foster healthy development from the very first days of life.

Acknowledgment

The author acknowledges using Perplexity AI for assistance with rephrasing and generating some sections of the text, specifically for language refinement and idea clarification.

Author details

Elaunire Monica Agianipe[1]*, Ndep Antor Odu[2], Akpan Margaret Inemiesit[2], Undie Emmanuel Ugbong[1] and Efut Joseph Ajah[2]

1 College of Nursing Sciences, Obudu, Cross River State, Nigeria; Department of Nursing Sciences, Havilla University, Nde, Ikom, Cross River State, Nigeria

2 Department of Public Health, University of Calabar, Calabar, Cross River State, Nigeria

*Address all correspondence to: abuamonique@gmail.com

References

[1] Herlihy JM, Shaikh A, Mazimba A, Gagne N, Grogan C, Mpamba C, Sooli B, Simamvwa G, Mabeta C, Shankoti P, Messersmith L, Semrau K, Hamer DH. Local perceptions, cultural beliefs and practices that shape umbilical cord care: A qualitative study in Southern Province, Zambia. PloS One. 2013;**8**(11): e79191. DOI: 10.1371/journal.pone.0079191

[2] World Health Organization. Newborn mortality. 2024. https://www.who.int/news-room/fact-sheets/detail/newborn

[3] Wenani D, Burgoine K, Williams SL, Musaba M, Gebrmichael T, Clarke A, Blanks KJH, Nantale R, Nawanga J, Kiguli S, English M, Waiswa P, Darmstadt GL, Matovu JKB, Mukunya D. Perceptions, beliefs, and current practices regarding neonatal skin care and emollient use in eastern Uganda: A qualitative study. BMC Pediatrics. 2023;**23**:223. DOI: 10.1186/s12887-023-04040-y

[4] Wogabaga J, Burgoine K, Kakuru A, Nambozo A, Chebet M, Tumuhamye J, Wanume B, Oguttu F, Musaba M, Napyo., Wani S, Olupot-Olupot P, QWeeks AD, Tylleskär T, Mukunya. Incidence and risk factors for clinical omphalitis among neonates in Eastern Uganda using chlorhexidine gel for cord care: A community-cohort study. BMC Pediatrics. 2025;**25**:55. DOI: 10.1186/s12887-025-05428-8

[5] UNICEF. Neonatal death. 2025. https://data.unicef.org/topic/child-survival/neonatal-mortality/

[6] Chlohexidine working group. *Implementing the World Health Organization Revised Recommendations on Cord Care*. Country guidance for umbilical cord care. 2018

[7] Duru CO, Oyeyemi AS, Adesina AD, Nduka I, Tobin-West C, Nte A. Sociocultural practices surrounding newborn cord care in Bayelsa State, Nigeria. PLOS Global Public Health. 2023;**3**(3):e0001299. https://pmc.ncbi.nlm.nih.gov/articles/PMC10047526/

[8] Abegunde D, Orobaton N, Beal K, Bassi AP. Trends in newborn umbilical cord care practices in Sokoto and Bauchi States of Nigeria: The where, who, how, what and the ubiquitous role of traditional birth attendants: A lot quality assurance sampling survey. BMC Pregnancy and Childbirth. 2017;**17**:1. DOI: 10.1186/s12884-017-1551-x

[9] Anyakorah PE, Aguna FC, Innocent DC, Uwandu-Uzoma AC, Ekeleme UG, Obasi CC, Eneh SC, Ahunam CP, Dike IC, Maduekwe VC, Ayando OD, Duruji CO, Innocent RC, Uwaezuoke PC, Adenuga OO, Emerole CO. A qualitative systematic review of umbilical cord care practices in Nigeria. BMC Pediatrics. 2025;**25**(1):34. DOI: 10.1186/s12887-025-05387-0

[10] Wogabaga J, Burgoine K, Kakuru A, Nambozo B, Chebet M, Tumuhamye J, Wanume B, Oguttu F, Musaba MW, Napyo A, Wani S, Olupot-Olupot P, Weeks AD, Tylleskär T, Mukunya D. Incidence and risk factors for clinical omphalitis among neonates in Eastern Uganda using chlorhexidine gel for cord care: A community-cohort study. BMC Pediatrics. 2025;**25**(1):55. DOI: 10.1186/s12887-025-05428-8.

[11] Ans M, Hussain M, Ahmed F, Khan K, Abbas S, Sultan M. Umbilical cord

care practices and cord care education of Mothers attending health care (Pakistan Prospect). Health. 2023;**15**:20–32. DOI: 10.4236/health.2023.151002

[12] Wright J, Umar-Farouk O, Ricca J. Scale-up of chlorhexidine for umbilical cord care in Nigeria. Usaid. 2017

[13] Gelano TF, Bacha YD, Abate D. Effect of chlorhexidine cord application on prevention of Neonatal Sepsis In Developing Countries: Systematic review and meta-analysis. International Journal of Health Sciences(Qassim). 2029;**13**(1):40–51

[14] Abua MA, Odu NA, Madubuattah LC, Ogunkola IO. Cultural patterns and outcomes of umbilical cord care among caregivers in Africa: A systematic review. Annals of Medicine and Surgery. 2023;**85**:3553–3562. https://pmc.ncbi.nlm.nih.gov/articles/PMC10328678/

Chapter 6

Navigating Caregiving and Work: Key Psychosocial Predictors of Quality of Life Amidst Familism in Japan's Evolving Long-Term Care System

Hiromi Nakamura-Thomas and Nobuyuki Sano

Abstract

Supporting family caregivers is critical for sustainable long-term care systems globally. Family caregivers often experience compromised psychological well-being due to limited social participation and caregiving distress. While diverse psychosocial supports exist internationally, establishing culturally congruent interventions is paramount, particularly in East Asian societies where family caregiving disproportionately impacts women amidst strong familism. Japan faces a unique challenge in 2025 as all baby boomers reach age 75, intensifying the need for their children to balance caregiving with social participation. This chapter explores innovative psychosocial support strategies for working adult caregivers in Japan to maintain their long-term care-related quality of life, integrating considerations of familism, cultural norms, and the evolving long-term care system to foster more resilient caregiving pathways. For this aim, we identified key psychosocial predictors of the long-term care-related quality of life in working family caregivers.

Keywords: psychosocial support, family caregivers, quality of life, familism, cultural norms

1. Introduction

Family caregivers of older adults often experience compromised psychological well-being due to caregiving distress and limited social participation [1–4]. In Japan, the long-term care insurance system, launched in 2000, was intended to shift the responsibility of elder care from the family to society [5]. Despite this, the system continues to rely heavily on informal care. Nearly half (46%) of the four million community-living care recipients receive assistance from coresiding family members, with another 12% receiving care from relatives living elsewhere, all in addition to formal services [6].

This reliance on family creates an acute challenge as Japan approaches 2025, the year when all its baby boomers will be over age 75 [7]. This demographic shift intensifies the pressure on the working-age generation to balance demanding careers with caregiving responsibilities. A key goal of Japan's long-term care system is to maintain the quality of life (QoL) of all involved [8]. However, with no established strategy for maintaining the QoL of family caregivers, there is an urgent need to develop effective psychosocial supports. To achieve this, we must first identify the key factors that influence the QoL of working family caregivers in Japan.

2. The Adult Social Care Outcomes Toolkit

The World Health Organization (WHO) defines QoL as an individual's perception of their life within their cultural context, considering their goals and concerns [9]. To measure this specifically within a care context, the Adult Social Care Outcomes Toolkit (ASCOT) was developed in the United Kingdom. The ASCOT is designed to measure Social Care-Related Quality of Life (SCRQoL), the aspects of life that are impacted by long-term care needs and services [10, 11]. The ASCOT has several versions, including one for informal caregivers (ASCOT-Carer) [10] and one for community-dwelling care recipients [11].

While initially developed for economic evaluation [12], ASCOT is now primarily valued for its ability to capture a holistic view of an individual's QoL [13]. A previous UK-based study has shown that ASCOT-Carer scores are significantly correlated with key psychosocial factors, including the caregiver's motivations, perceived autonomy, feelings of loneliness, positive and negative reactions to caregiving, the quality of their relationship with the care recipient, and overall satisfaction with official long-term care services for their care recipients. ASCOT-Carer scores are also significantly correlated with health-related QoL [14]. Notably, one's reason for caregiving was a significant predictor of SCRQoL. For example, caregivers who cited "having time because of not working or working part-time" reported higher ASCOT-Carer scores [15], highlighting a potential conflict between full-time employment and caregiver well-being. While ASCOT has proven useful in Western contexts, its applicability to Japan requires careful consideration due to cultural and systemic differences, as discussed below.

3. The Japanese landscape: Familism and the working caregiver

The context of informal caregiving in Japan differs significantly from that of Western nations, where the ASCOT-Carer was developed. In many European countries, financial support is provided to individuals offering informal care, leading to the categorization of "informal paid caregivers" [10]. Moreover, broader definitions of "informal caregiver" (including friends and acquaintances) exist [10]. This heterogeneity in defining informal care underscores the importance of studies employing the ASCOT-Carer to clearly delineate between paid and unpaid caregivers, as well as between family caregivers and the wider group encompassing friends. In contrast, Japan offers minimal formal support for working caregivers, with caregiving leave limited to five days annually per care recipient.

Most importantly, caregiving for frail or ill relatives is deeply viewed as a family matter, a responsibility that cultural norms and familism – a value system rooted in

Confucianism – often place on younger female relatives [16, 17]. This disproportionate burden is reflected in health outcomes; informal caregiving adversely affects female family caregivers' mental health and life satisfaction, but not that of male family caregivers [18]. This cultural backdrop makes it critical to understand whether findings from UK-based studies are applicable to Japan. The existing research faces three key limitations in the Japanese context. The first limitation is socio-cultural differences in long-term care systems and caregiving norms. The second limitation is the lack of validated Japanese versions for many psychosocial measures used in previous ASCOT studies. The third limitation is methodological constraints, as prior analyses using simple correlations may not capture the interwoven nature of psychosocial variables.

Given these challenges, this chapter seeks to uncover the psychosocial determinants of caregiver well-being in Japan, using ASCOT-Carer as a lens and employing a robust analytical approach tailored to the complexity of caregiving experiences.

4. Clarifying key concepts

This section clarifies the key concepts used throughout the chapter to ensure a common understanding.

4.1 Social Care-Related Quality of Life (sSCRQol)

SCRQoL refers to the aspects of an individual's QoL that are considered important and are potentially affected by adult social care services. Although this concept was originally developed to assess the well-being of community-dwelling care recipients, it has since been adapted to evaluate the experiences of informal caregivers, acknowledging that caregiving responsibilities can significantly influence their own QoL. In this chapter, SCRQoL is assessed using the ASCOT-Carer instrument, which is specifically designed to capture these multidimensional aspects of informal caregivers' lives.

4.2 Adult Social Care Outcomes Toolkit (ASCOT)

The ASCOT is a suite of instruments designed to measure SCRQoL. These tools are specifically for adults living in the community who receive care, as well as their informal caregivers. The ASCOT-Carer includes domains such as occupation, control over daily life, personal safety, and social participation, allowing for a multidimensional assessment of caregiver well-being. In this chapter, the ASCOT-Carer instrument is employed to evaluate the SCRQoL of informal family caregivers.

5. Methods

5.1 Research approach and design

The primary aim of this chapter was to identify key psychosocial predictors of SCRQoL in working family caregivers. Identifying these factors is a critical first step toward developing effective strategies to support the QoL in this population.

Building on previous research that found associations between the ASCOT-Carer score and various psychosocial factors [14, 15], we hypothesized that a set of interwoven variables would predict caregiver SCRQoL. The key factors selected for our model were loneliness, reactions to caregiving, relationship quality, social support, psychological well-being and distress, satisfaction with official services, motivation for caregiving, and the culturally specific concept of IKIGAI (a sense of life worth living).

A research study of community-dwelling care recipients in Japan successfully used a large sample (n = 1,141) to model predictors such as self-rated health, financial worries, satisfaction with official services, and official care need level [19]. To ensure sufficient statistical power for testing the complex relationships in the current study's model, a comparably large sample was deemed necessary. Therefore, we aimed to recruit 1,500 working family caregivers. The following sections provide a detailed justification for the inclusion of each factor, grounded in existing literature and the Japanese cultural context.

5.2 Justification of variable selection

5.2.1 IKIGAI (sense of a life worth living)

IKIGAI, a concept rooted in Japanese culture, was employed as a key variable. It has been shown to decrease psychological burden in family caregivers [20] and has demonstrated significant relationships with well-being and depression among people in England [21]. It was specifically included to reflect cultural values and to serve as a proxy for caregiver motivations, as other applicable questionnaires for a Japanese context were unavailable.

5.2.2 Loneliness

Loneliness is a critical factor, as research indicates it directly and indirectly impacts caregiver stress [22, 23]. It is frequently observed in caregivers and is significantly associated with anxiety, depression, and overall health decline [24–26].

5.2.3 Positive and negative reactions to caregiving

Family caregivers often experience a mix of positive and negative reactions. Negative reactions, such as schedule disruptions and a sense of having "no choice," are linked to psychological distress and even abusive behaviors, while positive experiences are associated with a greater sense of responsibility [27–29].

5.2.4 Relationship quality

The quality of the relationship between the caregiver and care recipient can significantly influence the caregiving experience. High relationship quality is linked to lower subjective burden and higher satisfaction [30], whereas significant time commitments (e.g., 80 + hours/month) can damage the relationship [31]. However, some studies have found no link between relationship cohesion and caregiver burden [32].

5.2.5 Psychological well-being and distress

The emotional toll of caregiving is well-documented, with many family caregivers reporting emotional strain, depression, and higher rates of chronic illness [33]. While some research finds no significant differences in depression by race/ethnicity, cultural beliefs and stigma can create barriers to seeking help, making this a crucial factor to consider [34, 35].

5.2.6 Social support

The structure and composition of a caregiver's social network are vital for providing support. People selectively draw on their network for specific needs [36, 37]. Stronger perceived social support and robust social networks are associated with lower caregiving burden and better self-rated health [38, 39]. Social support positively contributes to reducing feelings of loneliness, although it does not directly or positively contribute to mental health in Japanese adults [40].

5.2.7 Motivation for caregiving

The motivation for taking on the caregiving role is a significant predictor of caregiver outcomes, including SCRQoL and strain [41]. For instance, caregivers who perceive a greater sense of choice in their role are more likely to continue providing care [42]. Furthermore, the quality of a caregiver's motivation correlates with their well-being, a relationship that is influenced by factors such as their perceived competence, autonomy, and the quality of their relationship with the care recipient [43].

5.2.8 Satisfaction with official services

Previous research among unpaid informal caregivers in the UK found a significant correlation between their ASCOT-Carer scores and their satisfaction with official services provided for them and their care recipients [14]. Furthermore, service satisfaction has been shown to significantly predict caregiver stress in other populations, such as mothers of children with autism [44]. Therefore, examining the predictive role of service satisfaction specifically in the context of working family caregivers is a crucial step for informing both users and providers of long-term care services.

5.3 Sampling and inclusion criteria

Participants for this chapter were recruited based on five specific inclusion criteria. Individuals were required to be: (1) employed in a paid role (i.e., a working caregiver), (2) providing care for a community-dwelling family member who was officially registered as a care recipient under Japan's long-term care insurance system, (3) providing care for a duration of more than one month, (4) a primary family caregiver, and (5) unpaid for their family caregiving duties. This final criterion is noteworthy as it reflects the context of Japan at the time, where a national financial support system for family caregivers was not in place.

5.4 Data collection

5.4.1 Participant recruitment and procedure

Data for this study were collected online between September 1st and 7th, 2025. The sample was drawn from a panel of 5,189 registered working family caregivers managed by *Intage* Inc., a major research and crowdsourcing firm in Japan (https://www.intage.co.jp). From this panel, participants were randomly recruited nationwide across all 47 prefectures (Japan's local governments), with the sampling stratified by population density to ensure geographic representation. The firm's academic survey department then posted information about the survey to the selected panelists aged 18–65. This age range was selected to correspond with Japan's legal age of adulthood (18) and the statutory retirement age (65).

Potential participants first reviewed a description of the study. Consent was obtained when they voluntarily opted-in to begin the survey. An initial screening ensured that all participants met the inclusion criteria outlined previously. Those who qualified were then directed to the main response page containing the set of questionnaires.

5.4.2 Measures

The online survey included the following validated instruments to test the hypothetical model.

5.4.2.1 ASCOT-Carer

the validated Japanese version of the ASCOT-Carer, a measure for SCRQoL in family caregivers, was used [45]. The Japanese version retains the same structural components as the original version, such as the seven attributes and four response options. The seven attributes are occupation (doing things with value and enjoyment), control over daily life, looking after oneself, personal safety, social participation and involvement, space and time to be oneself, and feeling supported and encouraged. For each attribute, there are four possible response options representing a continuum of outcome states from best to worst: "ideal state," "no needs," "some needs," and "high-level needs." Scores are calculated using Japanese-specific preference weights and range from 0.02 to 1.00, with higher scores indicating better SCRQoL [46].

5.4.2.2 IKIGAI-9

The validated IKIGAI scale with nine items (IKIGAI-9) was used to measure this concept [47]. It assesses positive emotions, future orientation, and the meaning of one's existence. Items are rated on a 5-point scale (1 = not applicable at all to 5 = well applicable), with total scores ranging from 9 to 45. Higher scores represent a stronger sense of IKIGAI.

5.4.2.3 The 3-item Revised UCLA Loneliness Scale

The 3-item Revised UCLA Loneliness Scale for Japanese (R-UCLA-3-J) was employed to measure loneliness [48]. Participants rated how often they felt they lacked companionship, felt left out, or felt isolated on a 3-point Likert scale (1 = hardly ever to 3 = often). Scores range from 3 to 9, with higher scores indicating greater loneliness.

5.4.2.4 The 10-item Caregiver Reaction Assessment

The Japanese version of the 10-item Caregiver Reaction Assessment (CRA-10-J) was used to measure positive and negative reactions to caregiving [49]. Items are rated on a 5-point scale (1 = not agree at all to 5 = totally agree). The total score ranges from 10 to 50, with higher scores indicating a greater level of caregiving burden.

5.4.2.5 The 4-item Relationship Rewards Scale

The 4-item Relationship Rewards Scale (RRS-4) was used to measure relationship quality [50]. The scale was previously implemented with the original ASCOT-Carer [14]. Items (e.g., feeling happy with the relationship) were rated on a 4-point scale (0 = never to 3 = always). After reverse-scoring one item, the total score ranges from 0 (lowest relationship reward) to 12 (highest relationship reward).

5.4.2.6 WHO-5 Well-Being Index

The WHO-5 Well-Being Index for Japanese was used to measure psychological well-being [51]. This index focuses on subjective positive well-being. It consists of five items rated on a 6-point scale (0 = at no time to 5 = all of the time). The raw score ranges from 0 (worst possible well-being) to 25 (best possible well-being).

5.4.2.7 Kessler 6 (K6)

the K6 scale for the Japanese version was also used to measure psychological distress [52]. This scale focuses on general psychological distress. It consists of six items rated on a 5-point scale (0 = none of the time to 4 = all of the time). The total score ranges from 0 (no distress) to 24 (highest distress).

5.4.2.8 Social support scale

this chapter employed a social support scale developed for Japanese adults. This scale includes perceptions of both the provision and acceptance of social support. The responses did not differ between densely populated and rural areas. It has four question items with Yes or No response alternatives [53]: (1) I obtain emotional support, (2) I wish to offer emotional support, (3) I obtain instrumental support, and (4) I wish to offer instrumental support.

5.4.2.9 Motivation for caregiving

To measure the motivation for caregiving, this chapter used a list of common reasons identified specifically for Japanese family caregivers in a recent rapid review [54]. Participants were asked to select all applicable motivations from the following options: “Because of the wish of the care recipient,” “Less expensive than using nursing homes," "Sufficient support (formal and informal) is available," "My own benefits and/or rewards (e.g., perceiving positive feelings)," and "Others."

5.4.2.10 Satisfaction with official services

To measure satisfaction with official services, we adapted an approach from previous research that used the original ASCOT-Carer [14], employing a five-point scale (1 = extremely dissatisfied to 5 = extremely satisfied). This approach was chosen because, while no single standardized measurement exists, the importance of capturing service satisfaction is gaining international attention [55–57]. Ensuring that long-term care services meet the needs of users – including both care recipients and their family caregivers – is considered essential for system sustainability and for upholding human rights.

5.4.3 Demographic and caregiving variables

Participants provided detailed information about their personal, work, and caregiving situations. The specific variables and their corresponding response options are detailed below. A "do not want to indicate" option was available for most personal items.

5.4.3.1 Personal information

Personal information included participants' sex, age, education, financial worries, and the presence of chronic health conditions. Participants selected from "man," "woman," or "do not want to indicate" for their sex. Participants were asked to enter their age as a number. They selected their highest level of education from "high school," "vocational school/junior college after high school," "university," or "postgraduate school" for their education. Participants chose the option that best described their financial situation: "no worry," "a little bit worried," "a lot of worries," or "overwhelming worries" for their financial worries. For their marital status, response options were "married," "never married," "divorcee," or "widow or widower." For the presence of chronic health conditions, participants were asked if they had any chronic health conditions requiring medical follow-up, with the options "yes" or "no."

5.4.3.2 Work-related information

Work-related information included participants' employment style and annual income (Million Japanese Yen). For their employment style, response options included "full-time employee," "part-time employee," "entrepreneur," or "executive board member." Participants selected their income bracket from "below 1," "1 to 3," "3 to 6," "6 to 9," "9 to 12," "12 to 20," or "20 and more" for their annual income.

5.4.3.3 Caregiving context

Caregiving context included coresidence with their primary care recipient, the number of care recipients, and the reasons for providing care. Participants were asked if they resided with their primary care recipient, with "yes" or "no" as response options for the coresidence question. They were also asked to enter the number of people they provided care for. Regarding the reasons for providing care, justifying the inclusion of this variable is important.

5.4.4 Primary care recipient information

Primary care recipient information included their sex, age, relationship to the participants, and official care need level. For the care recipient's sex, response options were "man," "woman," or "do not want to indicate." Participants were asked to enter the care recipient's age as a number. Participants identified who the primary care recipient was from the options: "own mother," "own father," "spouse," "mother-in-law," "father-in-law," "grandparent," "child and/or grandchild," "sibling," or "others." Participants selected the recipient's official care need level under Japan's long-term care system: "low (more independent)," "moderate," "high (heavily dependent)," or "don't know."

5.5 Data analysis

The data analysis was conducted through a multi-step process. The initial stages involved descriptive statistics and preliminary analyses to summarize the data, evaluate the psychometric properties of the scales, and select variables. The final stage was a multiple linear regression analysis to identify predictors of the ASCOT-Carer score. Data were analyzed using IBM Statistical Package for the Social Sciences (SPSS Statistics) version 29.0.0.0 (IBM, Chicago, IL, USA) for Japanese and HAD (version 18), a software package that includes these nonparametric tests [58].

5.5.1 Stage 1: Descriptive statistics and psychometric evaluation

First, descriptive statistics were calculated to summarize the basic characteristics of the participants and their care recipients (as detailed in Section 3.4.3). Descriptive statistics for the total scores of all measures (ASCOT-Carer and others) were also calculated, including the range, median, mean, standard deviation, skewness, and kurtosis. To assess the internal consistency of the attachment scale specifically, both Cronbach's alpha and McDonald's omega were computed. A value above 0.78 for Cronbach's alpha and 0.81 for McDonald's omega was expected [59].

Second, the psychometric properties of the scales were evaluated. This involved examining the response distributions for each ASCOT-Carer item and calculating inter-item Pearson's correlation coefficients. The correlation coefficients were interpreted using the following thresholds: limited (0.00–0.25), fair (0.25–0.50), moderate (0.50–0.75), or excellent (0.75–1.0) [60].

5.5.2 Stage 2: Variable selection and final regression model

Third, preliminary bivariate analyses were conducted to inform the final model. Spearman's correlation coefficients were computed between the ASCOT-Carer score and all other measures to assess the strength of their relationships and to screen for potential multicollinearity. The coefficients were interpreted as limited (0.00–0.25), fair (0.25–0.50), moderate (0.50–0.75), or excellent (0.75–1.0) [60].

Fourth, group comparisons were performed to identify significant demographic and situational variables. The ASCOT-Carer scores were compared across groups using the *Brunner–Munzel* test (for two groups) and the *Kruskal–Wallis H* test (for multiple groups). Variables that showed a significant association in these tests were selected for inclusion in the final model.

Finally, a multiple linear regression analysis was performed. The predictor variables included the total scores from the psychosocial measures and the significant demographic/situational variables identified in the previous step. As a key diagnostic, multicollinearity was formally assessed using the variance inflation factor (VIF) and tolerance statistics, which are the reciprocal of the VIF (1 - the coefficient of determination: R^2). Following established guidelines, VIF values greater than 5 and tolerance values lower than 0.2 were considered indicative of problematic multicollinearity [61].

5.6 Ethical consideration

This survey received ethical approval from the institutional review board at Saitama Prefectural University (No. 2025–082). All procedures were conducted in accordance with the Declaration of Helsinki. The recruitment firm provided potential participants with a detailed explanation of the survey and its privacy policy. Participants indicated their initial agreement to provide information by proceeding to the survey. Before final submission, their informed consent was reconfirmed by asking them to verify their voluntary participation. As compensation for their time, participants received reward points from the firm, which could be redeemed for products. To ensure anonymity, the final data set provided by the firm did not include any personal identifiers, such as registration numbers or email addresses.

6. Results

A total of 1,619 working family caregivers completed the survey. Participants were drawn from all 47 prefectures (Japan's local governments), with the sample stratified by population density to ensure geographic representation. The average time for survey completion was 16 minutes, and no missing data were detected in the final dataset.

6.1 Descriptive statistics and psychometric evaluation

Table 1 details the participants' personal and work-related information, caregiving context, and their care recipients' information. The sample consisted of 865 men (53%) and 754 women (47%), with an age range of 19–65 years. The largest age group was 50–59 years (45%), followed by 60–65 years (29%). In terms of education, 40% had graduated from a university. Regarding their financial worries, one-third of participants reported having "a little worry" (33%), "a lot of worries" (29%), and "overwhelming worries" (26%). The participants were nearly evenly split between married individuals (43%) and those who were single with no marriage history (41%). Just over half (54%) of the participants reported having chronic health conditions.

Regarding their employment style, 56% were full-time employees, followed by part-time employees (28%). Nearly 38% of the participants chose three to six million Japanese yen as their annual income.

Most participants (73%) resided with their primary care recipient, and the vast majority (86%) cared for a single individual. For their motivations for caregiving

Variable		%
Personal information		
Sex	Men	53.43
	Women	46.57
	Do not want to indicate	0
Age group (years old)	19–29	2.35
	30–39	6.18
	40–49	17.54
	50–59	45.03
	60–65	28.91
	Do not want to indicate	0
Education	High school	28.10
	Vocational school/junior college	24.83
	University	40.27
	Postgraduate school	5.25
	Do not want to indicate	1.54
Financial worries	No worry	8.03
	A little worry	33.48
	A lot of worries	29.15
	Overwhelming worries	25.51
	Do not want to indicate	3.83
Marital status	Married	42.80
	Never married	40.58
	Divorcee	12.54
	Widow/widower	1.98
	Do not want to indicate	2.10
The presence of a chronic health condition	Yes	54.29
	No	42.62
	Do not want to indicate	3.09
Work-related information		
Employment style	Full-time employee	56.33
	Part-time employee	27.86
	Entrepreneur	11.43
	Executive board member	4.39

Variable			%
Annual income (million Japanese yen)	Below 1		2.10
	1–3		12.48
	3–6		27.79
	6–9		16.37
	9–12		10.32
	12–20		0.24
	20 and more		2.16
	I don't know		10.25
	Do not want to indicate		12.29
Caregiving context			
Coresidence	Yes		73.13
	No		26.87
	Do not want to indicate		0
Number of care recipients	1		86.04
	2		12.29
	3 and more		1.67
Motivations for caregiving (Multiple answers)	Wish of the care recipient		51.27
	Less expensive than nursing homes		37.68
	Sufficient support is available		34.47
	My own benefits/rewards		28.91
	Others		3.27
	Do not want to indicate		6.86
Social support	I obtain emotional support	Yes	51.27
		No	48.73
	I wish to offer emotional support	Yes	37.68
		No	62.32
	I obtain instrumental support	Yes	34.47
		No	65.53
	I wish to offer instrumental support	Yes	28.91
		No	71.09
Satisfaction with official services	Extremely satisfied		6.24
	Satisfied		34.40
	Neither satisfied nor dissatisfied		36.26
	Dissatisfied		15.07
	Extremely dissatisfied		8.03
Care recipients' information			
Sex	Men		27.49
	Women		72.51
	Do not want to indicate		0

Variable		%
Age group (years old)	2–17	0.43
	18–64	6.36
	65–74	8.40
	75–100	84.81
Kinship to caregiver	Own mother	63.87
	Own father	20.51
	Spouse	4.82
	Mother-in-law	3.77
	Father-in-law	1.73
	Grandparent	2.10
	Child/grandchild	1.79
	Sibling	0.74
	Others	0.68
*Official care need level**	Low	62.08
	Moderate	17.11
	High	12.66
	Don't know	8.15

*Note: *care need level in the long-term care system in Japan.*

Table 1.
Participants' personal and work-related information, caregiving context, and care recipients' information (1,619 working family caregivers with no missing data).

(multiple answers allowed), the most common response was "wish of the care recipient" (51%), followed by it being "less expensive than using nursing homes" (38%). Regarding their social support, 51% of them obtained emotional support, and 38% wished to offer emotional support. Regarding their satisfaction with official services, 36% of them chose "neither satisfied nor dissatisfied." More than 40% of them perceived satisfaction ("extremely satisfied" or "satisfied"), while more than 23% perceived dissatisfaction ("extremely dissatisfied" or "dissatisfied").

Regarding the primary care recipients, most were women (73%) and were aged 75 or older (85%). The most common kinship to the participants was their own mother (64%), followed by their own father (21%). Regarding the official care need levels, 62% were classified as "low" (interpreted to be more independent), while 17% were "moderate" and 13% were "high" (interpreted to be less independent and needing significant help with self-care).

The response distribution for each ASCOT-Carer item is presented in **Figure 1**. The most frequent response option across the attributes was "no need," ranging from 43% to 61%. For the attribute of "occupation," the response options "no need" (39%) and "some needs" (40%) were nearly equal in frequency.

Table 2 presents the descriptive statistics for the total scores of all measures. The scores for each measure fell within their expected ranges. Notably, some participants scored the highest possible scores, while others scored above the established clinical cutoffs on certain scales. The internal consistency for all scales was adequate, with

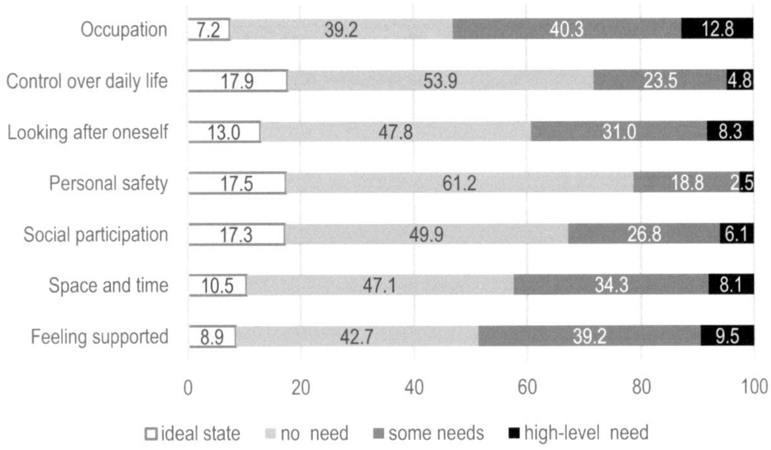

Figure 1.
Response characteristics by question item and response options in the ASCOT-Carer (%) (1,619 working family caregivers with no missing data).

Measure	Score	MED	MEA	SD	SKE	KUR	α	ω
ASCOT-Carer	0.022–1.000	0.73	0.67	0.25	−0.58	−0.76	0.85	0.88
IKIGAI-9	9–45	24	24.16	7.47	0.31	0.03	0.92	0.92
R-UCLA-3	3–9	8	5.50	1.87	0.30	−0.80	0.85	0.86
K6	0–24	8	8.32	6.22	0.64	−0.21	0.94	0.94
CRA-10	10–50	31	31.22	7.17	−0.00	−0.04	0.86	0.86
WHO-5	0–25	9	10.01	5.72	0.53	−0.19	0.93	0.93
RRS-4	4–12	8	8.49	2.10	−0.04	−0.36	0.83	0.85

Note: ASCOT-Carer = Adult Social Care Outcomes Toolkit for informal caregivers, R-UCLA-3 = The 3-item Revised UCLA Loneliness Scale, K6 = The Kessler 6 scale, CRA-10 = the 10-item Caregiver Reaction Assessment, WHO-5 = WHO5 Well-Being Index, RRS-4 = the 4-item Relationship Rewards Scale, MED = Median, MEA = Mean, SD = Standard Deviation, SKE = Skewness, KUR = Kurtosis, α = Cronbach's Alpha, ω = McDonald's Omega, n.a. = not applicable.

Table 2.
Descriptive statistics of the measures (1,619 working family caregivers with no missing data).

Cronbach's alpha values ranging from 0.83 to 0.94, and McDonald's omega values ranging from 0.85 to 0.94.

Table 3 presents the interitem correlation coefficients in the ASCOT-Carer. Correlation coefficients were at fair to moderate levels (all $p < 0.001$).

7. Variable selection and regression modeling

Preliminary analyses were conducted to identify variables significantly associated with the ASCOT-Carer score. As shown in the correlation matrix in **Table 4**, the scores on the psychosocial measures were correlated with the ASCOT-Carer score at fair to moderate levels (all $p < 0.001$).

Variable	1	2	3	4	5	6	7
1. Occupation	1.000						
2. CON	0.556*	1.000					
3. LOK	0.569*	0.532*	1.000				
4. PER	0.418*	0.362*	0.400*	1.000			
5. SOC	0.414*	0.378*	0.385*	0.469*	1.000		
6. SPA	0.641*	0.506*	0.587*	0.475*	0.556*	1.000	
7. FEE	0.523*	0.400*	0.454*	0.399*	0.551*	0.610*	1.000

Note: CON = control over daily life, LOO = looking after oneself, PER = personal safety, SOC = social participation and involvement, SPA = space and time to be oneself, FEE = feeling supported and encouraged.
$^*p$ <0.001

Table 3.
Interitem correlation coefficients in the ASCOT-Carer (1,619 working family caregivers with no missing data).

Measure	1	2	3	4	5	6	7
1	1.000						
2	0.583*	1.000					
3	-0.567*	-0.464*	1.000				
4	-0.577*	-0.471*	0.672*	1.000			
5	-0.605*	-0.524*	0.499*	0.567*	1.000		
6	0.688*	0.629*	-0.498*	-0.573*	-0.502*	1.000	
7	0.401*	0.365*	-0.372*	-0.420*	-0.534*	0.402*	1.000

Note: 1 = Adult Social Care Outcomes Toolkit for informal caregivers, 2 = IKIGAI-9, 3 = The 3-item Revised UCLA Loneliness Scale, 4 = The Kessler 6 Scale, 5 = the 10-item Caregiver Reaction Assessment, 6 = the 4-item Relationship Rewards Scale, 7 = the WHO-5 Well-Being Index.
$^*p$ <0.001

Table 4.
Correlation matrices of scores between measures (1,619 working family caregivers with no missing data).

As shown in **Table 5**, significant differences in ASCOT-Carer scores were found across several demographic groups, including age group, financial worries, marital status, and the presence of chronic health conditions. Pairwise comparisons revealed that caregivers aged 60–65 had significantly higher scores than those aged 40–49 (adjusted p = 0.001) and 50–59 (adjusted p <0.001).

In financial worries, caregivers with "overwhelming worries" scored significantly lower than all other groups (all adjusted p <0.001). Those with "a lot of worries" scored lower than those with "no worry" or "a little worry" (both adjusted p <0.001).

In marital status, caregivers with no marital history scored significantly lower than married caregivers (adjusted p <0.001). Regarding the presence of chronic health conditions, caregivers with "do not want to indicate" scored significantly lower than those with no chronic health condition (p = 0.007). No significant differences in scores were found between groups divided based on caregiver sex or education level.

Variable		%	Descriptive statistics in the score			Group comparison			Pairwise caparisons (adjusted *p*-value)
			MED	Mean	SD	*BM* or *H* value	*df*	*p*-value	
Sex	Men	53.43	0.738	0.674	0.258	0.609	1	0.543	
	Women	46.57	0.709	0.670	0.245				
Age group (years old)									
	1. 19–39	8.53	0.810	0.693	0.289	32.866	3	<0.001	2 & 4 (0.001), 3 & 4 (<0.001)
	2. 40–49	17.54	0.669	0.642	0.271				
	3. 50–59	45.03	0.673	0.646	0.248				
	4. 60–65	28.91	0.810	0.725	0.225				
Education									
	High school	28.10	0.709	0.662	0.257	4.342	4	0.362	
	VSJC	24.83	0.724	0.684	0.238				
	University	40.27	0.745	0.678	0.255				
	POST	5.25	0.672	0.652	0.277				
	DNW	1.54	0.553	0.606	0.198				
Financial worries									
	1. No worry	8.03	0.910	0.831	0.200	331.832	4	<0.001	4 & 1 (<0.001), 4 & 2 (<0.001), 4 & 3 (<0.001), 4 & 5 (<0.001), 3 & 1 (<0.001), 3 & 2 (<0.001)
	2. A little	33.48	0.857	0.776	0.191				
	3. A lot of	29.15	0.709	0.664	0.233				
	4. OVE	25.51	0.492	0.500	0.255				
	5. DNW	3.83	0.683	0.650	0.252				
Marital status									
	1. Married	42.80	0.779	0.706	0.245	28.593	4	<0.001	1 & 2 (0.001)
	2. NEV	40.58	0.666	0.640	0.256				
	3. Divorcee	12.54	0.751	0.666	0.256				
	4. WW	1.98	0.783	0.719	0.249				
	5. DNW	2.10	0.587	0.623	0.219				
The presence of chronic health conditions									
	1. Yes	54.29	0.709	0.660	0.256	13.992	2	0.001	1 & 2 (0.014), 1 & 3 (0.033), 2 & 3 (0.007)
	2. No	42.62	0.765	0.695	0.244				
	3. DNW	3.09	0.573	0.580	0.265				

Note: MED = median, SD = standard deviation, BM = Brunner–Munzel test, H = Kruskal–Wallis H test, df = degree of freedom, VSJC = vocational school/junior college, POST = postgraduate school, DNW = do not want to indicate, OVE = overwhelming worries, NEV = never married, WW = widow/widower.

Table 5.
Group comparisons of the ASCOT-Carer scores according to the of the caregivers' personal information.

Table 6 details the comparisons for work-related characteristics. A significant difference was observed based on employment style. Pairwise comparisons indicated that "executive board members" had significantly higher scores than both "full-time" and "part-time" employees (both adjusted $p = 0.001$). No significant difference was found between groups divided based on annual income.

Comparisons related to the caregiving context are presented in **Table 7**. Caregivers who resided with their primary care recipient had significantly lower scores than caregivers who did not ($p < 0.001$).

Variable	%	Descriptive statistics in the score			Group comparison			Pairwise caparisons (adjusted *p*- value)
		MED	Mean	SD	*H* value	*df*	*p*-value	
Employment style								
1. FTE	56.33	0.726	0.668	0.258	14.490	3	0.002	1 & 4 (0.001), 2 & 4 (0.001)
2. PTE	27.86	0.704	0.668	0.241				
3. ENT	11.43	0.714	0.672	0.245				
4. EBM	4.39	0.910	0.762	0.254				
Annual income (Million Japanese yen)								
0–3	14.58	0.699	0.630	0.269	10.061	4	0.039	
3–6	27.79	0.754	0.690	0.242				
6–9	16.37	0.726	0.684	0.242				
9 +	12.72	0.760	0.678	0.273				
DNK	22.54	0.692	0.665	0.240				

Note: MED = median, SD = standard deviation, H = Kruskal–Wallis H test, df = degree of freedom, FTE = full-time employee, PTE = part-time employee, ENT = entrepreneur, EBM = executive board member, 9 + = 9 and more, DNK = do not know.

Table 6.
Group comparisons of the ASCOT-Carer scores according to variables of the caregivers' work-related information.

Variable	%	Descriptive statistics in the score			Group comparison			Pairwise caparisons (adjusted *p*- value)
		MED	Mean	SD	BM or H value	*df*	*p*-value	
Coresidence								
Yes	73.13	0.704	0.659	0.254	3.22	1	<0.001	
No	26.87	0.804	0.709	0.242				
Number of care recipients								
1	86.04	0.727	0.676	0.249	1.048	1	0.296	
2 and more	13.96	0.702	0.650	0.271				

Variable		%	Descriptive statistics in the score			Group comparison			Pairwise caparisons (adjusted *p*- value)
			MED	Mean	SD	BM or H value	*df*	*p*-value	
Motivations for caregiving (multiple answers)									
WIS	Y	51.27	0.715	0.665	0.250	1.558	1	0.119	
	N	48.73	0.745	0.681	0.254				
LES	Y	37.68	0.703	0.651	0.259	2.719	1	0.007	
	N	62.32	0.738	0.685	0.247				
SUF	Y	34.47	0.784	0.705	0.246	4.019	1	<0.001	
	N	65.53	0.699	0.655	0.254				
MYO	Y	28.91	0.829	0.738	0.239	7.483	1	<0.001	
	N	71.09	0.679	0.646	0.239				
Social support									
OES	Y	64.98	0.824	0.750	0.216	20.142	1	<0.001	
	N	35.02	0.520	0.528	0.250				
WES	Y	73.56	0.795	0.714	0.237	12.212	1	<0.001	
	N	26.44	0.543	0.555	0.255				
OIS	Y	48.05	0.845	0.767	0.208	16.761	1	<0.001	
	N	51.95	0.593	0.585	0.257				
WIS	Y	79.99	0.775	0.704	0.239	10.427	1	<0.001	
	N	20.01	0.530	0.546	0.265				
Satisfaction with official services									
1. ES		6.24	0.970	0.918	0.127	535.51	4	<0.001	1 & 2 (<0.001), 1 & 3 (<0.001), 1 & 4 (<0.001), 1 & 5 (<0.001), 2 & 3 (<0.001), 2 & 4 (<0.001), 2 & 5 (<0.001), 3 & 4 (<0.001), 3 & 5 (<0.001), 4 & 5 (<0.001)
2. Satisfied		34.40	0.910	0.796	0.187				
3. NSD		36.26	0.650	0.639	0.220				
4. Dissatisfied		15.07	0.520	0.537	0.225				
5. EDS		8.03	0.286	0.355	0.248				

Note: MED = median, SD = standard deviation, BM = Brunner–Munzel test, H = Kruskal–Wallis H test, df = degree of freedom, WIS = wish of the care recipient, LES = less expensive than the use of nursing homes, SUF = sufficient support (formal and informal), MYO = my own benefits/rewards, Y = Yes, meaning choosing it, N=No, meaning not choosing it, OES = I obtain emotional support, WES = I wish to offer emotional support, OIS = I obtain instrumental support, WIS = I wish to offer instrumental support, ES = extremely satisfied, NSD = neither satisfied nor dissatisfied, EDS = extremely dissatisfied.

Table 7.
Group comparisons of the ASCOT-Carer scores according to variables of the caregiving context.

In motivations for care giving, caregivers who cited "sufficient support available" ($p < 0.001$) or "my own benefits and/or reward" ($p < 0.001$) as motivations for caregiving had significantly higher scores than those who did not cite these reasons.

In social support, caregivers who cited "I obtain emotional support," "I wish to offer emotional support," "I obtain instrumental support," or "I wish to offer instrumental support" had significantly higher scores than those who did not cite these reasons.

Regarding satisfaction with official services, all pairwise comparisons showed significant differences in the ASCOT-Carer scores (all adjusted $p < 0.001$). Caregivers who indicated "extremely satisfied" had significantly higher scores than other groups. Caregivers who indicated "satisfied" had significantly higher scores than those who indicated "neither satisfied nor dissatisfied," "dissatisfied," or "extremely dissatisfied." Caregivers who indicated "neither satisfied nor dissatisfied" had significantly higher scores than those who indicated "dissatisfied" or "extremely dissatisfied." Caregivers who indicated "dissatisfied" had significantly higher scores than those who indicated "extremely dissatisfied."

No significant difference was found between groups divided based on the number of care recipients (one individual or two or more individuals), or motivation for caregiving according to the "wish of the care recipient" or "less expensive than the use of nursing homes."

Table 8 details the comparisons for the primary care recipients' information. Pairwise comparisons revealed that caregivers of recipients with a "low" care need level had significantly higher scores than those caring for recipients with "moderate" (adjusted $p = 0.003$) or "high" (adjusted $p < 0.001$) care need levels. No significant score difference was found between groups divided based on the care recipients' sex, age groups, or kinship.

For a more precise variable selection for the regression model, several significant demographic variables were recategorized into broader groups. For instance, responses of "I do not know" and "I do not want to indicate" were treated as missing data for this step. Age was collapsed into "older" (60–65) and "middle-aged"

Variable	%	Descriptive statistics in the score			Group comparison			Pairwise caparisons (adjusted *p*-value)
		MED	Mean	SD	*BM* or H value	*df*	*p*-value	
Care recipients' sex								
Men	27.49	0.731	0.673	0.270	0.713	1	0.176	
Women	72.51	0.718	0.672	0.245				
Age group (years old) in care recipients								
2–17	0.43	0.325	0.325	0.219	9.212	3	0.027	
18–64	6.36	0.804	0.804	0.265				
65–74	8.40	0.726	0.726	0.270				
75–100	84.81	0.724	0.742	0.249				
Kinship to caregivers								
Own mother	63.87	0.730	0.668	0.270	2.619	2	0.270	
Own father	20.51	0.714	0.670	0.244				
Others	15.62	0.757	0.689	0.260				

Variable	%	Descriptive statistics in the score			Group comparison			Pairwise caparisons (adjusted *p*-value)
		MED	Mean	SD	*BM* or H value	*df*	*p*-value	
Official care need level in care recipients*								
1. Low	62.08	0.771	0.700	0.241	29.824	3	<0.001	
2. Moderate	17.11	0.676	0.637	0.262				1 & 2 (0.003),
3. High	12.66	0.603	0.605	0.273				1 & 3 (<0.001)
4. DNK	8.15	0.654	0.643	0.247				

Note: MED = median, BM = Brunner–Munzel test, H = Kruskal–Wallis H test, df = degree of freedom.
**Care need level in the long-term care system in Japan, DNK = do not know.*

Table 8.
Group comparisons of the ASCOT-Carer scores according to variables of the primary care recipient's information.

(40–59). In financial worries, three groups were recategorized as follows: "no worry or a little worry," "a lot of worries," and "overwhelming worries." In marital status, two groups were recategorized as follows: "married caregivers" and "never married caregivers." In official care need level, two groups were recategorized as follows: "low" and "moderate or high" care need levels.

As shown in **Table 9**, the score comparisons using these new categories confirmed the previous findings. For example, older caregivers had significantly higher scores than middle-aged caregivers ($p < 0.001$).

Regarding financial worries, a significant difference was detected. Pairwise comparisons confirmed that caregivers with "overwhelming worries" had significantly lower scores than those with "no worry or a little worry" (adjusted $p < 0.001$) or those with "a lot of worries" (adjusted $p < 0.001$). Caregivers with "a lot of worries" had significantly lower scores than those with "no worry or a little worry" (adjusted $p < 0.001$).

In marital status, married caregivers had significantly higher scores than those who never married ($p < 0.001$). Care givers of recipients with a "low" care need level had significantly higher scores than those caring for recipients with a "moderate or high" level ($p < 0.001$).

A multiple linear regression analysis with a stepwise method was conducted, resulting in three distinct models presented in **Table 10**. Those models were robust, explaining a significant portion of the variance (adjusted $R^2 > 0.63$) and showing no issues with multicollinearity (all VIF <2.5, and all tolerance values >0.40).

The specific predictors for each model are outlined below. For Model 1, eight variables emerged as significant predictors. The selected predictors were higher psychological well-being (WHO-5; $\beta = 0.282$, $p < 0.001$), higher satisfaction with official services ($\beta = 0.271$, $p < 0.001$), lower negative reactions to caregiving (CRA-10; $\beta = -0.204$, $p < 0.001$), lower psychological distress (K6; $\beta = -0.144$, $p < 0.001$), lower loneliness (UCLA Loneliness Scale; $\beta = -0.100$, $p < 0.001$), and the perception of obtaining emotional social support ($\beta = 0.088$, $p < 0.001$). Additionally, a "low" care need level in the care recipients ($\beta = 0.060$, $p = 0.002$) and citing "sufficient support" as a caregiving motivation ($\beta = 0.056$, $p = 0.006$) were also significant predictors of higher scores.

Variable (valid sample)	%	Descriptive statistics in the score			Group comparison			Pairwise caparisons (adjusted *p*-value)
		MED	Mean	SD	*BM* or H value	*df*	*p*-value	
Age groups (1,619)								
Old	*31.60*	0.810	0.725	0.225	5.466	1	<0.001	
Middle	*68.40*	0.673	0.645	0.254				
Financial worries (1,557)								
1. NW	43.16	0.875	0.786	0.194				1 & 2 (<0.001),
2. A lot of	30.31	0.709	0.664	0.233	319.046	2	<0.001	1 & 3 (<0.001),
3. OVE	26.53	0.492	0.500	0.255				2 & 3 (<0.001)
Marital status (1,350)								
Married	51.33	0.779	0.706	0.245	4.291	1	<0.001	
NEV	48.67	0.666	0.640	0.256				
Official care need level(1,487)*								
Low	67.59	0.771	0.700	0.241	4.628	1	<0.001	
M/H	32.41	0.652	0.623	0.267				

Note: MED = Median, BM = Brunner–Munzel test, H = Kruskal–Wallis H test, df = degree of freedom; age groups: old = aged 60–65, middle = aged 40–59; NW=no worry and a little worry, OVE = overwhelming worries, NEV = never married. *Care need level in the long-term care system in Japan, M/H = moderate and high care need levels.

Table 9.
Group comparisons of the ASCOT-Carer scores according to variables with group category revisions.

For Model 2, seven variables were extracted as significant predictors. The selected predictors were higher well-being (WHO-5; $\beta = 0.288$, $p < 0.001$), higher satisfaction with services ($\beta = 0.221$, $p < 0.001$), lower psychological distress (K6; $\beta = -0.146$, $p < 0.001$), lower negative reactions to caregiving (CRA-10; $\beta = -0.134$, $p < 0.001$), and the perception of obtaining emotional support ($\beta = 0.090$, $p < 0.001$). Lower loneliness (UCLA Loneliness Scale; $\beta = -0.095$, $p = 0.001$) and a "low" care need level ($\beta = 0.058$, $p = 0.003$) were also significant.

For Model 3, nine variables were identified as significant predictors. The predictors were higher well-being (WHO-5; $\beta = 0.264$, $p < 0.001$), higher satisfaction with services ($\beta = 0.217$, $p < 0.001$), lower negative reactions to caregiving (CRA-10; $\beta = -0.188$, $p < 0.001$), lower psychological distress (K6; $\beta = -0.111$, $p < 0.001$), lower loneliness (UCLA Loneliness Scale; $\beta = -0.109$, $p < 0.001$), the perception of obtaining emotional support ($\beta = 0.087$, $p < 0.001$), and a "low" care need level ($\beta = 0.065$, $p < 0.001$). Finally, a higher score on the IKIGAI-9 scale ($\beta = 0.073$, $p = 0.001$) and citing "sufficient support" as a caregiving motivation ($\beta = 0.045$, $p = 0.005$) were also significant predictors of higher ASCOT-Carer scores.

8. Discussion

This chapter explored key psychosocial predictors of SCRQoL in working family caregivers, representing a first attempt to inform effective support strategies for this population.

Variable	*Unstandardized coefficients* B	Standardized coefficients *β*	*p*-value	VIF	Tolerance values
Model 1 ($R = 0.796$, $R^2 = 0.633$, adjusted $R^2 = 0.630$, $F = 204.714$, $p < 0.001$, $n = 958$)					
WHO-5	0.012	0.282	<0.001	1.799	0.556
Satisfaction	0.055	0.217	<0.001	1.421	0.704
CRA-10	-0.007	-0.204	<0.001	1.819	0.550
K6	-0.006	-0.144	<0.001	2.461	0.456
R-UCLA-3	-0.013	-0.100	<0.001	2.210	0.452
SS1	0.046	0.088	<0.001	1.303	0.767
OCNL	0.033	0.060	0.002	1.009	0.991
SUF	0.029	0.056	0.006	1.039	0.963
Model 2 ($R = 0.794$, $R^2 = 0.630$, adjusted $R^2 = 0.627$, $F = 231.219$, $p < 0.001$, $n = 958$)					
WHO-5	0.013	0.288	<0.001	1.786	0.560
Satisfaction	0.056	0.221	<0.001	1.416	0.706
K6	-0.005	-0.146	<0.001	2.463	0.406
CRA-10	-0.007	-0.134	<0.001	2.428	0.454
R-UCLA-3	-0.013	-0.095	0.001	2.202	0.454
SS1	0.048	0.090	<0.001	1.301	0.769
OCNL	0.032	0.058	0.003	1.008	0.992
Model 3 ($R = 0.769$, $R^2 = 0.633$, adjusted $R^2 = 0.631$, $F = 283.615$, $p < 0.001$, $n = 1{,}417$)					
WHO-5	0.012	0.264	<0.001	2.016	0.496
Satisfaction	0.054	0.217	<0.001	1.410	0.709
CRA-10	-0.007	-0.188	<0.001	1.848	0.451
K6	-0.004	-0.111	<0.001	2.323	0.431
R-UCLA-3	-0.015	-0.109	<0.001	2.211	0.452
SS1	0.046	0.087	<0.001	1.332	0.751
IKIGAI-9	0.002	0.073	0.001	1.967	0.508
OCNL	0.035	0.065	<0.001	1.016	0.984
SUF	0.024	0.045	0.005	1.040	0.961

Note: VIF = variance inflation factor, WHO-5 = The WHO-5 Well-Being Index, Satisfaction = satisfaction with official services (1 = extremely dissatisfied, 2 = dissatisfied, 3 = neither satisfied nor dissatisfied, 4 = satisfied, 5 = extremely satisfied), CRA10 = the 10-item Caregiver Reaction Assessment, K6 = the Kessler 6 scale, R-UCLA-3 = the 3-item Revised UCLA Loneliness Scale, SS1 = obtaining emotional social support (1 = no, 2 = yes), OCNL = Official care need level for care recipient (1 = moderate or high care need levels, 2 = low care need level), SUF = sufficient support (formal and informal) for motivation for caregiving (1 = no, 2 = yes).

Table 10.
Predictors of the ASCOT-Carer score in working family caregivers.

8.1 Summary and interpretation of key findings

A key finding was the identification of several consistent predictors of higher SCRQoL. Across all models, these included higher psychological well-being, greater satisfaction with official services, lower negative reactions to caregiving, lower psychological distress, and less loneliness. Other significant factors included obtaining emotional support, a lower care need level in the recipient, perceiving sufficient support as a motivation for caregiving, and a higher sense of IKIGAI. These findings support our initial hypotheses and are consistent with previous ASCOT-Carer studies conducted in the UK [14, 15].

Interestingly, no model selected the care recipient's personal factors (sex and age) or the quality of the caregiver-recipient relationship as significant predictors. This suggests that future support strategies should focus primarily on the caregivers' own perceptions and psychological states, as these may be effective across different care recipient demographics and relationship dynamics.

The significance of cultural norms was also highlighted. In countries with caregiving values rooted in Confucianism, working family caregivers are particularly vulnerable as they balance family responsibilities with workforce participation [5–8]. While familism can be a protective factor, our findings suggest that potential support strategies must be culturally congruent, addressing not only practical burdens but also the caregivers' perceptions of purpose, sacrifice, and obligation [62].

8.2 The central role of social support

Social support emerged as a particularly critical factor. Although there is no standardized measure for social support specific to Japanese working family caregivers, this study used existing methods to demonstrate its importance. "Obtaining emotional support" was a consistent predictor in all three models, and "availability of sufficient support" was a significant motivator linked to higher SCRQoL. This aligns with the "feeling supported and encouraged" domain of the ASCOT-Carer itself and reinforces previous findings on the power of social support to buffer psychological distress in family caregivers [63–66].

Similarly, satisfaction with services was a strong predictor of SCRQoL. This finding may reflect the importance of service quality, which includes factors like accessibility, provider attitude, and cost-effectiveness. Future studies should aim to disentangle these components to identify which aspects of service quality have the greatest impact on caregiver SCRQoL.

8.3 Implications for practice and future research

The findings have clear implications. Previous studies have shown that psychosocial and behavioral interventions can improve the QoL for caregivers of individuals with cancer, dementia, and amyotrophic lateral sclerosis [67–72]. Our results suggest that similar strategies, tailored to working family caregivers and focused on enhancing well-being, reducing loneliness, and bolstering social support, should be developed. Crucially, the effectiveness of these new interventions should be evaluated using the ASCOT-Carer to measure changes in SCRQoL. Future research should also aim to identify the specific types and qualities of social support that are most effective at easing psychological distress in this population.

8.4 Limitations

While this chapter provides valuable insights, several limitations should be considered. Firstly, some measures, like IKIGAI-9 and the Japanese version of the

Caregiver Reaction Assessment (CRA-10-J), are culture-specific, meaning the selected predictors may not be directly applicable to caregivers in other cultures. Secondly, the findings are based on the service model of the Japanese long-term care system and may not generalize to countries with different service structures. Thirdly, the participants were exclusively family caregivers, so the findings may not extend to paid caregivers or those caring for friends and acquaintances. Lastly, participants were recruited from a single crowdsourcing firm, and their characteristics may differ from caregivers who are not registered with this or any similar firm.

9. Conclusion

This chapter successfully identified key psychosocial predictors of SCRQoL in working family caregivers. The results underscore that higher SCRQoL is strongly associated with a combination of caregivers' internal resources and external support systems. Key internal factors included higher psychological well-being, lower psychological distress, fewer negative reactions to caregiving, less loneliness, and a stronger sense of IKIGAI. Crucially, external factors like higher satisfaction with official services and the perception of emotional and practical support were also powerful predictors. These findings provide a vital evidence base for developing concrete and effective strategies to support the QoL for this important population.

Acknowledgments

The authors wish to thank all the family caregivers who participated in this chapter. We also acknowledge the contributions of the crowdsourcing firm that assisted with data collection.

Funding information

This research was supported by a grant from Saitama Prefectural University.

Conflict of Interest

The authors declare no potential conflicts of interest with respect to the research, authorship, and/or publication of this article.

Author details

Hiromi Nakamura-Thomas[1*] and Nobuyuki Sano[2]

1 Graduate School of Health, Medicine and Welfare, School of Health, Medicine and Welfare, Saitama Prefectural University, Koshigaya, Japan

2 Faculty of Medical Sciences, Fukuoka International University of Health and Welfare, Fukuoka, Japan

*Address all correspondence to: nakamura-hiromi@spu.ac.jp

References

[1] Vlachantoni A, Feng Z, Wang N, Evandrou M. 2020. Social participation and health outcomes among caregivers and no caregivers in Great Britain. Journal of Applied Gerontology. **39** (12):1313–1322. DOI: 10.1177/0733464819885528

[2] Smith T, Saunders A, Heard J. 2020. Trajectory of psychosocial measures amongst informal caregivers: Case-controlled study of 1375 informal caregivers from the english longitudinal study of ageing. Geriatrics (Basel). **5**(2):26. DOI: 10.3390/geriatrics5020026

[3] Zhao X, Liu H, Fang B, Zhang Q, Ding H, Li T. 2021. Continuous participation in social activities as a protective factor against depressive symptoms among older adults who started high-intensity spousal caregiving: Findings from the China health and retirement longitudinal survey. Journal of Mental Health and Aging. **25**(10):1821–1829. DOI: 10.1080/13607863.2020.1822283

[4] Barbosa FCS, Delerue Matos AM, Voss GDS, Eiras AFS. 2022. The importance of social participation for life satisfaction among spouse caregivers aged 65 and over. Health and Social Care in the Community. **30** (5):e3096–e3105. DOI: 10.1111/hsc.13754

[5] Ministry of health, labour and welfare. An outline of the long-term care system. Tokyo: Ministry of Health, Labour and Welfare; 2022. (in Japanese). Available from: https://www.mhlw.go.jp/content/000801559.pdf [Accessed: 2024-April-1]

[6] Ministry of Health, Labour and Welfare. A survey of circumstances of primary informal family caregivers. Tokyo: Ministry of Health, Labour and Welfare; 2022. (in Japanese). Available from: https://www.mhlw.go.jp/toukei/saikin/hw/k-tyosa/k-tyosa22/dl/05.pdf [Accessed: 2023-April-1]

[7] Cabinet Office. Chapter One: Ageing Population. Tokyo:Cabinet Office;2020 (in Japanese). Available from https://www8.cao.go.jp/kourei/whitepaper/w-2020/html/zenbun/s1_1_1 [Accessed: 2024-April-1]

[8] Ministry of Health, Labour and Welfare. A proposal for ideal systems for provision of medicine and long-term care after 2025. Tokyo: Ministry of Health, Labour and Welfare; 2023. (in Japanese). Available from: https://www.mhlw.go.jp/content/12403550/001059091.pdf [Accessed: 2024-April-1]

[9] WHO. WHOQOL: Measuring quality of life. Available from: https://www.who.int/tools.whoqol [Accessed: 2024-April-1]

[10] Rand S, Malley J, Netten A, Forder JE. Factor structure and construct validity of the adult social care outcomes toolkit for carers (ASCOT-Carer). Quality of Life Research. 2015;**24**:26012614. DOI: 10.1007/s11136-015-1011-x

[11] Netten A, Burge P, Malley J, Potoglou D, Towers AM, Bzazier J, et al. Outcomes of social care for adults: Developing a preference-weighted measure. Health Technology Assessment. 2012;**16**:1–166

[12] Batchelder L, Malley J, Burge P, Lu H, Saloniki EC, et al. Carer social care-related quality of life outcomes: Estimating English preference weights for the adult social care outcomes toolkit for carers. Value in Health. 2019;**22**(12):1427–1440. DOI: 10.1016/j.jval.2019.07.014

[13] Bulamu NB, Kaambwa B, Ratcliffe J. A systematic review of instruments for measuring outcomes in economic evaluation within aged care. Health and Quality of Life Outcomes. 2015;**13**:179. DOI: 10.1186/s12955-015-0372-8

[14] Rand S, Malley J, Vadean F, Forder J. Measuring the outcomes of long-term care for unpaid carers: Comparing the ASCOT-Carer, Carer Experience Scale and EQ-5D-3L. Health and Quality of Life Outcomes. 2019;**17**:184. DOI: 10.1186/s12955-019-1254-2

[15] Rand S, Malley J, Forder J. 2018. Are reasons for care-giving related to carers' care-related quality of life and strain? Evidence from a survey of carers in England. Health and Social Care in the Community. **27**(1):151–160. DOI: 10.1111/hsc.12634

[16] Hofstede G. Culture Consequences: Comparing Values, Behaviors, Institutions and Organizations across Nations. California: Sage; 2001

[17] Yoo WK.A research methodology for Korean neo-confucianism. Acta Koreana. 2013;**16**(1):177–197

[18] Le DD, Ibuka Y. Understanding the effects of informal caregiving on health and well-being: Heterogeneity and mechanisms. Social Science and Medicine. 2023;**317**:115630. DOI: 10.1016/j.socscimed.2022.115630

[19] Moriyama Y, Morikawa M, Nakamura-Thomas H, Shiroiwa T, Tamiya N, Takahashi H. Measurement of social care related quality of life among elderly people with long-term care needs using the Japanese version of the Adult Social Care Outcomes Toolkit (ASCOT). Journal of the National Institute of Public Health. 2020; In Japanese with an English abstract **69**(5):460–470

[20] Okamoto K, Harasawa Y. 2009. Predictor of increase in caregiver burden for disabled elderly at home. Archives of Gerontology and Geriatrics. **49**(1):129–131. DOI: 10.1016/j.archger.2008.06.001

[21] Fido D, Kotera Y, Asano K. English translation and validation of the Ikigai-9 in a UK Sample. International Journal of Mental Health and Addiction. 2019;**1**:8. DOI: 10.1007/s11469-019-00150-w

[22] Peavy G, Mayo AM, Avalos C, Rodriguez A, Shifflett B, Edland SD. Perceived stress in older dementia caregivers: Mediation by loneliness and depression. American Journal of Alzheimer's Disease and Other Dementias. 2022;**37**:15333175211064756. DOI: 10.1177/15333175211064756

[23] Victor CR, Rippon I, Quinn C, Nelis SM, Martyr A, Hart N, Lamont R, Clare L. The prevalence and predictors of loneliness in caregivers of people with dementia: Findings from the IDEAL programme. Aging and Mental Health. 2021;**7**:1232–1238. DOI: 10.1080/13607863.2020.1753014

[24] Guan Z, Poon AWC, Zwi A. 2023. Social isolation and loneliness in family caregivers of people with severe mental illness: A scoping review. American Journal of Community Psychology. **72**(3-4):443–463. DOI: 10.1002/ajcp.12698

[25] Jabbari J, Pitzer KA, White Makinde K, Benson JJ, Demiris G, Oliver DP, Washington KT. 2024. Loneliness, psychological distress, and the moderating effect of positive aspects of caregiving among cancer caregivers. Supportive Care in Cancer. **32**(7):404. DOI: 10.1007/s00520-024-08599-9

[26] Chukwuorji JC, Amazue LO, Ekeh OH. 2017. Loneliness and psychological health of orthopaedic patients' caregivers: Does gender make a difference? Psychology, Health and Medicine. **22**(4):501–506. DOI: 10.1080/13548506.2016.1173711

[27] Aloweni F, Doshi K, Fook-Chong S, Malhotra R, Østbye T. 2019. The types of caregiving reactions experienced by the older spouse caregivers. Journal of Clinical Nursing. **28**(23-24):4538–4548. DOI: 10.1111/jocn.15044

[28] Wang M, Sun H, Zhang J, Ruan J. 2019. Prevalence and associated factors of elder abuse in family caregivers of older people with dementia in central China cross-sectional study. International Journal of Geriatric Psychiatry. **34**(2):299–307. DOI: 10.1002/gps.5020

[29] Hou D, Chen YX, He D, Zhang X, Fan X. 2020. The relationship between caregiver reactions and psychological distress in family caregivers of patients with heart failure. Journal of Cardiovascular Nursing. **35**(3):234–242. DOI: 10.1097/JCN.0000000000000636

[30] Tough H, Brinkhof MW, Siegrist J, Fekete C. 2017. Subjective caregiver burden and caregiver satisfaction: The role of partner relationship quality and reciprocity. Archives of Physical Medicine and Rehabilitation. **98**(10):2042–2051. DOI: 10.1016/j.apmr.2017.02.009

[31] Kolodziej IWK, Coe NB, Van Houtven CH. 2022. The impact of care intensity and work on the mental health of family caregivers: Losses and gains. The Journals of Gerontology. Series B, Psychological Sciences and Social Sciences. **77**(Suppl_1):S98–S111. DOI: 10.1093/geronb/gbac031

[32] Wu CY, Skidmore ER, Rodakowski J. 2019. Relationship consensus and caregiver burden in adults with cognitive impairments 6 months following stroke. PM&R: The Journal of Injury, Function, and Rehabilitation. **11**(6):597–603. DOI: 10.1002/pmrj.12009

[33] Petrovic M, Gaggioli A. Digital mental health tools for caregivers of older adults-a scoping review. Frontiers in Public Health. 2020;**8**:128. DOI: 10.3389/fpubh.2020.00128

[34] Whitney RL, Bell JF, Kilaberia TR, Link BM, Choula RB, Reinhard SC, Young HM. 2023. Diverse demands and resources among racially/ethnically diverse caregivers. Ethnicity and Health. **28**(6):912–931. DOI: 10.1080/13557858.2023.2179022

[35] Hurley D, Swann C, Allen MS, Ferguson HL, Vella SA. 2020. A systematic review of parent and caregiver mental health literacy. Community Mental Health Journal. **56**(1):2–21. DOI: 10.1007/s10597-019-00454-0

[36] Wellman B. Wortley S different strokes from different folks: Community ties and social support. American Journal of Sociology. 1990;**96**:558–588

[37] Penning MJ. Receipt of assistance by elderly people: Hierarchical selection and task specificity. Gerontologist. 1990, **30**, 220–227

[38] Nemcikova M, Katreniakova Z, Nagyova I. Social support, positive caregiving experience, and caregiver burden in informal caregivers of older adults with dementia. Frontiers in Public Health. 2023;**11**:1104250. DOI: 10.3389/fpubh.2023.1104250

[39] Xian M, Xu L. 2020. Social support and self-rated health among caregivers of people with dementia: The mediating role of caregiving burden. Dementia (London). **19**(8):2621–2636. DOI: 10.1177/1471301219837464

[40] Toyoshima A, Sato S. Relationship between social support and mental health mediated by loneliness among the middle-age and elderly: An investigation using the UCLA Loneliness Scale Version 3. Ronen Shakai Gaku. 2013; in Japanese with an English abstract **35**(1):29–38

[41] Rand S, Malley J, Forder J. Are reasons for care-giving related to carers' care-related quality of life and strain? Evidence from a survey of carers in England. Health and Social Care in the Community. 2019;**27**:151–160. DOI: 10.1111/hsc.12634

[42] Pertl MM, Sooknarine-Rajpatty A, Brennan S, Robertson IH, Lawlor BA. Caregiver choice and caregiver outcomes: A longitudinal study of Irish spousal dementia caregivers. Frontiers in Psychology. 2019;**10**:1801. DOI: 10.3389/fpsyg.2019.01801

[43] Dombestein H, Norheim A, Lunde Husebø AM. 2020. Understanding informal caregivers' motivation from the perspective of self-determination theory: An integrative review. Scandinavian Journal of Caring Sciences. **34**(2): 267–279. DOI: 10.1111/scs.12735

[44] Fong VC, McLaughlin J, Schneider M. 2023. "We are exhausted, worn out, and broken": Understanding the impact of service satisfaction on caregiver well-being. Autism Research. **16**(11):2198–2207. DOI: 10.1002/aur.3024

[45] Nakamura-Thomas H, Yamaguchi M, Yamaguchi I, Rand S. Assessing the structural characteristics of the Japanese version of the adult social care outcomes toolkit for carers. Home Health Care Management and Practice. 2022;**34**:17–23. DOI: 10.1177/10848223211030269

[46] Shiroiwa T, Nakamura-Thomas H, Yamaguchi M, Morikawa M, Moriyama Y, Fukuda T, et al. Japanese preference weights of the adult social care outcomes toolkit for carers (ASCOT-carer). Quality of Life Research. 2022;**31**:2143–2151

[47] Imai T, Osada H, Nishimura Y. 2012. The reliability and validity of a new scale for measuring the concept of Ikigai (Ikigai-9. Japanese Journal of Public Health. **59**(7):433–439. DOI: 10.11236/jph.59.7_433

[48] Igarashi T. 2019. Development of the Japanese version of the three-item loneliness scale. BMC Psychology. **7**(1):20. DOI: 10.1186/s40359-019-0285-0

[49] Noguchi T, Nakagawa T, Jin X, Komatsu A, Togashi S, Miyashita M, Saito T. Development of a short form of the Japanese version of the Caregiver Reaction Assessment (CRA-J-10) among informal caregivers of older adults. Geriatrics and Gerontology

International. 2023. DOI: 10.1111/ggi.14824

[50] Williamson GM, Shaffer DR. Relationship quality and potentially harmful behaviors by spousal caregivers: How we were then, how we are now. Psychology and Aging. 2001;**16**:217–226. DOI: 10.1037/0882-7974.16.2.217

[51] Awata S, Bech P, Koizumi Y, Seki T, Kuriyama S, Hozawa A, et al. Validity and utility of the Japanese version of the WHO-Five Well-Being Index in the context of detecting suicidal ideation in elderly community residents. International Psychogeriatrics. 2007;**19** (1):77–88. DOI: 10.1017/s10416102060 04212

[52] Furukawa TA, Kawakami N, Saitoh M, Ono Y, Nakane Y, Nakamura Y, et al. The performance of the Japanese version of the K6 and K10 in the World Mental Health Survey Japan. International Journal of Methods in Psychiatric Research. 2008;**17**(3):152–158. DOI: 10.1002/mpr.257

[53] Saito Y, Kondo K, Yoshii S, Hirai H, Suemori K, Murata C, et al. Health and social support in older adults: Acceptance of provision. Koshu Eisei. 2005;**69**(8):661–665. in Japanese

[54] Sakakibara K, Katahira N. Literature review of the factors concerning continuing nursing care at home by family members. Nihon Zaitaku Care Gakkaishi. 2018; in Japanese with an English abstract **22** (1):114–122

[55] Lee AHI, Kang HY, Liu YA. 2021. A Pilot Study on the Satisfaction of Long-Term Care Services in Taiwan. International Journal of Environmental Research and Public Health. **19**(1):90. DOI: 10.3390/ijerph19010090

[56] Aung MN, Moolphate S, Aung TNN, Koyanagi Y, Kurusattra A, Chantaraksa S, Supakankunti S, Yuasa M. 2022. Effectiveness of a community-integrated intermediary care (CIIC) service model to enhance family-based long-term care for Thai older adults in Chiang Mai, Thailand: A cluster-randomized controlled trial TCTR20190412004. Health Research Policy and Systems. **20**(Suppl 1):110. DOI: 10.1186/s12961-022-00911-5

[57] Petrucha RRA, Hansen EG, Ironside LD, Lafrance OJM, Bryce RDT, Jacobson NA, Ramsden VR. 2022. Addressing the Long-Term Care Crisis: Identifying Opportunities for Improvement Using Rapid Reviews. Canadian Geriatrics Journal. **25**(1):79–87. DOI: 10.5770/cgj.25.535

[58] Shimizu H. An introduction to the statistical free software HAD: Suggestions to improve teaching, learning and practice data analysis. Journal of Media, Information and Communication. 2016;**1**: 59–73. in Japanese with an English abstract

[59] Zinbarg RE, Revelle W, Yovel I, Li W. 2005. Cronbach's α, Revelle's β, and Mcdonald's ω H: Their relations with each other and two alternative conceptualizations of reliability. Psychometrika. **70**(1):1–11. DOI: 10.1007/s11336-003-0974-7

[60] Munro BH. Statistical Methods for Health Care Research. Baltimore, MD, USA: Lippincott Williams & Wilkins; 2005

[61] Kim JH. 2019. Multicollinearity and misleading statistical results. Korean Journal of Anesthesiology. **72**(6): 558–569. DOI: 10.4097/kja.19087

[62] Falzarano F, Moxley J, Pillemer K, Czaja SJ. 2022. Family matters: Cross-cultural differences in familism and caregiving outcomes. The Journals of Gerontology: Series B. **77**(7):1269–1279. DOI: 10.1093/geronb/gbab160

[63] Sone T, Nakaya N, Tomata Y, Tsuji I. 2018. Risk of psychological distress in partners with functional disability among older Japanese adults. Geriatrics and Gerontology International. **18**(5):775–782. DOI: 10.1111/ggi.13254

[64] Ang S, Malhotra R. 2018. Expressive social support buffers the impact of care-related work interruptions on caregivers' depressive symptoms. Aging and Mental Health. **22**(6):755–763. DOI: 10.1080/13607863.2017.1317329

[65] Sandoval F, Tamiya N, Lloyd-Sherlock P, Noguchi H. 2019. The relationship between perceived social support and depressive symptoms in informal caregivers of community-dwelling older persons in Chile. Psychogeriatrics. **19**(6):547–556. DOI: 10.1111/psyg.12438

[66] Sánchez-Alcón M, Garrido-Fernández A, Cano-Rojas JM, Sánchez-Ramos JL, Ramos-Pichardo JD. 2024. Relationship between depressive symptoms, caregiver strain, and social support with dementia grief in family caregivers. Medicina (Kaunas). **60**(4):643. DOI: 10.3390/medicina60040643

[67] Gabriel I, Creedy D, Coyne E. 2020. A systematic review of psychosocial interventions to improve quality of life of people with cancer and their family caregivers. Nursing Open. **7**(5):1299–1312. DOI: 10.1002/nop2.543

[68] Song L, Qan'ir Y, Guan T, Guo P, Xu S, Jung A, Idiagbonya E, Song F, Kent EE. 2021. The challenges of enrollment and retention: A systematic review of psychosocial behavioral interventions for patients with cancer and their family caregivers. Journal of Pain and Symptom Management. **62**(3): e279–e304. DOI: 10.1016/j.jpainsymman.2021.04.019

[69] Lambert SD, Duncan LR, Culos-Reed SN, Hallward L, Higano CS, Loban E, Katz A, De Raad M, Ellis J, Korman MB, Sears C, Ibberson C, Walker L, Belzile E, Saha-Chaudhuri P, McTaggart-Cowan H, Peacock S. 2022. Feasibility, acceptability, and clinical significance of a dyadic, Web-based, psychosocial, and physical activity self-management program (TEMPO) tailored to the needs of men with prostate cancer and their caregivers: A multi-center randomized pilot trial. Current Oncology. **29**(2):785–804. DOI: 10.3390/curroncol29020067

[70] Guan T, Qan'ir Y, Conklin JL, Zimba CC, Bula A, Jumbo W, Wella K, Mapulanga P, Bingo SAM, Chilemba E, Haley J, Montano NP, Bryant AL, Song L. Systematic review of psychosocial interventions for adult cancer patients and their family caregivers in Sub-Saharan Africa. Global Public Health. 2023;**18**(1):2199062. DOI: 10.1080/17441692.2023.2199062

[71] Nasreen HE, Tyrrell M, Vikström S, Craftman Å, Syed Ahmad SAB, Zin NM, Aziz KHA, Mohd

Tohit NB, Md Aris MA, Kabir ZN. 2024. Caregiver burden, mental health, quality of life and self-efficacy of family caregivers of persons with dementia in Malaysia: Baseline results of a psychoeducational intervention study. BMC Geriatrics. **24**(1):656. DOI: 10.1186/s12877-024-05221-9

[72] Katz L, Gur A. 2024. Psychosocial intervention for family caregivers of ALS patients: A systematic review. Healthcare (Basel). **12**(12):1171. DOI: 10.3390/healthcare12121171

Chapter 7

Perspective Chapter: Moving Long-Term Care into Home, Community and Primary Healthcare Settings Amid Resource Constraints in Developing Nations

Emmanuel Edet Udontre

Abstract

This work underscores the urgent need for culturally sustainable, integrated health and social care systems for the promotion of healthy aging and a better quality of life for elders in developing nations. It reveals that the long-term care (LTC) system in developing and underdeveloped countries remains rudimentary, with elders relying on untrained family members and an under-resourced primary care system. The current reliance on costly, less-accepted residential care models and tertiary facilities must shift toward community-based solutions that promote aging in place, preserve dignity, and maintain independence. The aim of this work is to offer valuable insights into systemic gaps and propose the mainstreaming of agedcare into the home, community, and primary healthcare system framework because of its numerous merits. The key concepts, analysis, and positions presented in this paper provide evidence and robust ideas to stimulate discourse on policy direction and socio-economic planning that supports healthy aging and longevity despite scarce resources in developing nations. This work indicates that LTC of older persons at home, in the community, and in primary healthcare settings is not only preferred by most elders and families in developing nations but is also cost-effective and easy to integrate into already available care structures. The recommendations for consideration are the design of eldercare policies that support the integrated LTC model with home, community, and primary healthcare components; capacity development for care providers – gerontology nurses, personal support workers, social care workers, recreational therapists, among others; adequate funding of the primary healthcare system; and a focus on health promotion and disease prevention.

Keywords: moving, long-term care, homecare, primary healthcare system, resource constraints, developing nations

1. Introduction

Population aging is a positive development of the twentieth and twenty-first centuries, indicating an improvement in longevity better than previous eras, thanks to scientific innovation, improvements in health, education, socio-economic conditions, and reductions in fertility and mortality rates across the globe (World Health Organization [1]). By 2080, seniors who are 65 years or older will outnumber youths under 18 globally (United Nations Department of Economic and Social Affairs, UNDESA [2]). Aging of the population was first observed in the late nineteenth century when France and Sweden were noted as two countries where the number of persons aged 65 years and above rose to 7%, the benchmark then used to indicate an aging population (Rowland in Cook and Halsall [3]). France began experiencing population aging in 1865, and Sweden in 1890. Other countries experienced the graying of the population a bit later, such as the UK in 1930 and the United States of America in 1944. The Aging index, which is the ratio of elders aged 65 years or over to 100 youths aged 15 years or younger, is currently used as an indicator of population aging. It is projected that by 2030, countries in Europe will have aging index of 100, meaning there will be more elders than every 100 younger people aged 15 years and under in their population (National Research Council (US) Panel on a Research Agenda and New Data for an Aging World [4]). Experts in population studies and gerontology have repeatedly noted that although population aging began in developed nations in the middle of the twenty-first century, it has intensified in developing and less developed nations. In the next three decades, Africa, Asia, and Latin America – most of which are developing economically will be home to the largest population of elders (UNDESA [5]; Taylor and Powell [6]; UNDESA [7]). Some developing African and Asian nations have large populations with a significant segment of youths and young adults but are experiencing "gerontogrowth," indicating an increase in older persons aged 60 years and above in the population, with population aging approaching faster than some of these nations may imagine (Francisco [8]; Francisco [9]). Gerontogrowth and population aging are trends that call for a series of actions by governments, economic planners, health and agedcare system designers and managers, as well as families and communities. According to the World Health Organization (WHO) [10]; [11], at least 75% of older persons will need long-term care (LTC) at some point in their life course, including assistance from others to manage basic activities of daily living such as bathing, dressing, and eating. Moreover, globally, 142 million seniors (14% of the world population) living in 42 nations constitute the number whose LTC needs are unmet. An analysis of the above indicates the huge challenge facing developing nations amid their dwindling economic resources. The number of older persons aged 60 years and over in Africa in 2022 was about 78 million and is projected to more than double to about 165 million by 2050 for countries south of the Sahara (United Nations 2022 in World Bank [12]; WHO [13]). If 75% of the elders in Africa will need LTC, this means there are about 58 million elders currently, and in the next two decades, approximately over 123 million elders for whom the LTC system should be prepared to cater. According to the Asia Pacific Report on Population Aging 2022, the absolute number of older persons aged 60 years and over in Asia is approximately 469,000,000 and is expected to double to about 1.3 billion by 2050 (United Nations, Economic and Social Commission for Asia and the Pacific (ESCAP) (2022) [14]). Seventy-five percent (75%) of that number is approximately over 135 million, and by the next two decades, close to a billion. In most developing nations, the LTC system is either absent or rudimentary, and the primary healthcare system is very weak. As a result, the only available option is for hospitals to be utilized for acute, chronic, and LTC. However, the comprehensive LTC needs of older persons can hardly be met using this model. Therefore, developing nations should prepare LTC systems and structures, as well as the human resources, to care for about three-quarters of the population of older persons in their nations. This is without prejudice to the fact that the remaining 25% will still also need some services as senior citizens with full rights. The work involved in developing and sustaining LTC for these numbers of elders in middle- and low-income countries is enormous. As noted by WHO [15], Akingunola et al. [16], and Jeyasingam et al. [17], older persons utilize healthcare services more than younger persons. Many have more than one chronic ailment, consult multiple medical practitioners, and are on multiple medications. Some elders require multiple admissions due to acute conditions and need several follow-ups. This is against the backdrop that, although illness is not inherently part of the aging process and younger people can and do have chronic illnesses, noncommunicable diseases, multimorbidity, and comorbidities are more prevalent among older persons, hence the higher need for palliative and LTC. This is in addition to other physical, emotional, psychological, socio-economic, and spiritual needs.

The developed countries have responded to these needs by developing different formal, regulated LTC models, some of which have been in existence for decades and are constantly reviewed to improve their efficiency (Australian Government Department of Health, Disability and Ageing [18]; NHS England Digital - Adult Social Care Activity and Finance Report 2023–24 [19]). The Active Ageing Index (AAI), which indicates the capacity for older persons to lead active lives and contribute to socio-economic development, has continued to improve for most developed countries (United Nations Economic Commission for Europe [20]). The situation is not the same for most developing nations. The basic structures for LTC are unavailable. LTC of older persons is considered a responsibility of the family. Care is provided by informal, untrained carers, who are relatives, mainly young women, and the next facility for care is the hospitals – secondary and tertiary or specialty centers – which constitute the formal care setting. The primary healthcare system in most developing nations is weak, with inadequate staff and services. The community networks and support once relied upon have disintegrated. Family caregivers face material resource constraints, lack of caregiving knowledge, and opportunity costs such as missed education and employment opportunities. This reliance on family care perpetuates poverty and hinders socioeconomic development, especially for women and girls, and sometimes results in elder abuse and neglect.

The situation is succinctly stated by the WHO below:

> *Worldwide, the number of older people requiring care and support is increasing rapidly. At the same time, the proportion of younger people who might be able to provide this care is falling, and women, the traditional caregivers within many families, are already filling, or aspiring to, other social and economic roles. As a result, the assumption that families alone can meet the needs of older people with significant losses of capacity is outdated and neither sustainable nor equitable* (World Health Organization [13]).

In a captivating article, "Ageing in developing countries, who cares?", Thaver [21], drawing from his experience as a Professor of Community Health, vividly painted a picture of agedcare in a developing Asian country and concluded by noting that the challenge at hand in that nation is the increasing incidence of noncommunicable diseases and chronic ailments among senior citizens, leading to an increasing need for LTC. He further noted that the situation, though unaddressed appropriately, could have been better handled if there were strong advocates in the country who not only understood the magnitude of the challenge but also had the political clout to point out to policy makers, economic planners, and other stakeholders the cost-effective and viable solutions for implementation in order to promote healthy aging and a better quality of life. The above scenario is not far from what is occurring in most developing nations and rural communities of Africa, Asia, Latin America, and the Caribbean (World Bank [12], United Nations (ESCAP) [14], Cadmus, Adebusoye, Owoaje [22]). The writer, a gerontologist, gerontology nurse, and community/public health practitioner, having cared for older persons in clinical and community/public healthcare settings in and outside Africa and currently involved in building capacity in this field, was motivated when the opportunity arose to share some ideas on the above subject. This is an attempt toward advocate for the LTC of older persons using age-friendly environments, culturally acceptable, cost-effective, and sustainable models in resource-constrained settings. The main aim is to offer insights into systemic gaps in developing countries and propose the mainstreaming of agedcare into the home, community, and primary healthcare system framework because of its numerous merits in low-resource settings, such as proximity, acceptability, minimal cost for execution, support, and aging in place. It will also provide evidence and stimulate discourse on policy direction and socio-economic planning based on systems that support healthy aging and longevity in developing nations.

1.1 Long-term care

LTC "encompasses activities undertaken by others to ensure that those with a significant ongoing loss of physical or mental capacity can maintain a level of ability to be and to do what they have reason to value, consistent with their basic rights, fundamental freedoms, and human dignity" (WHO [23, 24]). LTC is defined as "a variety of ongoing health and social services provided for individuals who need assistance on a continuous basis because of physical or mental disabilities. Services can be provided in an institution, the home, or the community, and include informal services provided by professionals or agencies" (Institute of Medicine in Kar [25]). LTC involves services designed to meet, on a long-term basis, the health, physical, emotional, psychological, spiritual, personal, and social care needs of individuals. It is necessary to state at this point that LTC could be for individuals of any age, depending on their functional ability, health status, limitations, or disabilities. These could include children, adults living with disabilities, or older persons. The aim of LTC is to help individuals who need support to care for themselves live as independently and safely as possible. The point of need usually starts when the individual can no longer perform everyday activities on their own. However, this discourse is in the context of LTC for older persons. LTC for older persons focuses on care that meets the needs of seniors who cannot care for themselves independently. It is often referred to as agedcare, eldercare, senior care, gerontology care, or gerontology nursing. Nursing as a profession has tried to reduce the use of the term "geriatric nursing" and prefers "gerontology nursing" or "gerontology care" because it focuses on the comprehensive needs of older persons, which could include bio-physical, medical or health, social care, support services, housing and living arrangements, economic, and environmental support services, as opposed to being limited to just healthcare. The goal of LTC for older adults is the maintenance of healthy aging and the promotion of a better quality of life. This is a complex issue and not as straight forward as it appears. The bouquet of services must be provided by a multidisciplinary team through multisectoral collaboration (Touhy and Jett, 2014) [26]). The services and interventions could range from addressing physical, health, social, and spiritual needs, among others. A consistent and significant message from the field of aging over the years is that the above range of services cannot be achieved using the hospital setting alone but through a combination of various models, depending on the needs of individuals. When LTC facilities are used, it should be only when necessary. Moreover, no matter the models used, consideration should be given to the issues of quality, cost, acceptability, dignity, independence and autonomy, integration of care, and sustainability. Some developed countries that initially started with hospital-based LTC have reviewed, remodeled and moved to residential LTC and nursing home settings. Still, in these countries, there is a growing demand and shift to home and community care, as seen in Australia, Canada, China, Japan, and the UK (Australian Government Department of Health, Disability and Ageing [18]; Australian Institute of Health and Welfare [27]; Yue, Xiang, Li [28]; Ikegami [29]; Health and Social Services [30]). The questions that the governments of developing and underdeveloped nations should answer are: why are nations that experienced population aging over a century ago, and even some who had the experience more recently, opting for home and community-based agedcare services? Moreover, what model of LTC do older persons in developing countries prefer? Which model would be most culturally acceptable, affordable, and sustainable? Why did the concept of "aging in place" emerge? (Rosenwohl-Mack et al. [31]; Graybill et al. [32]). Largely, some studies have provided direction regarding various models, their merits, and demerits. When the issues of quality, client satisfaction, accessibility, acceptability, sustainability, dignity, autonomy, choice, individualized person-centered care, and integration of health and social care across the whole continuum of care along the life course are satisfied, among others, then that would be considered a good option (WHO [33,34] Gibson et al. [35]; Kok et al. [36]). In developing an LTC system that will be affordable, accessible, and sustainable, developing nations must bear the socio-economic dimensions in mind. Would it be better to build such a system around huge mega-structures that would only be sited in a few cities, or around already existing structures such as homes, primary healthcare facilities, and community centers? These nations should bear in mind that the aging trajectory is not really in favor of most elders. The aging process and the changes associated with it, though neither linear nor universal, depend on various extrinsic and intrinsic factors and cumulative advantages or disadvantages over the life course, putting elders in these regions at a socio-economic disadvantage (WHO [11]; Amarya et al. [37]). Thus, the type of LTC system that should be developed must be easy to use, close by, cheap, and convenient, to put it simply.

1.2 Developing and underdeveloped nations in context

In this paper, the World Economic Situation and Prospects (WESP) of 2024 criteria for the classification of countries was adopted (UNDESA [38]). WESP grouped the nations of the world into three categories: developed, emerging economies or economies in transition, and developing nations. The developing nations, based on the WESP classification, are countries in Africa, Eastern Asia (excluding Japan), Western and Southern Asia, Latin America, and the Caribbean. The per capita gross national income (GNI) is also used by WESP to divide nations into high-income, upper-middle-income, lower-middle-income, and low-income categories. In this discussion, reference to developing nations refers to lower-, middle-, and low-income countries, as well as developing and underdeveloped nations. Most developing nations are grappling with issues such as high infant and maternal mortality, poverty, economic instability, conflicts in some cases, weak health systems, the absence of or rudimentary agedcare systems, as well as the disintegration of family and community support networks. Eldercare is not being given adequate attention amid these various challenges (UNDP [39]; WHO [23]). These nations, though not identical, have socio-economic, geopolitical, and environmental circumstances that are not too far apart. Some, however, have made gigantic strides socio-economically in recent years.

2. Literature review

2.1 Aging and agedcare: Ancient yet with modern lessons

Aging, agedcare, gerontology, and geriatrics are ancient sciences with a modern history, offering numerous lessons for present and future generation(s). Starting from "Eugeria" or "successful ageing" of Aristotle, then "Gerocomie" or "the science of treatment of old people" of Celsus and Galen, to Geriatrics of Ignatz Nascher and Gerontology of Elie Metchnikoff, these fields have evolved significantly. From great foresight to the numerous biological, psychological, and social theories of aging, the lessons have been clear: the strength of youth will not remain the same in later life, but adjustment and resilience are possible. The message is aging is a process, a developmental stage in life, with benefits and potential if elders are adequately cared for to maintain their functional abilities. In the later years of life, the social and economic resources for some individuals may change, requiring that they be supported (Abdi et al. [40]). The lessons from the field of aging continue: older persons have general, specific, and varied needs, and they do not respond in the same way as youths and adults in health and illness, and so they deserve well-thought-out interventions. Aging can be "accelerated or decelerated" depending on the interplay of "positive and negative factors" as well as "intrinsic and extrinsic" phenomena and processes. Daily habits, nutrition, and activities can affect aging positively if healthy, and negatively if the reverse is the case (Haupt et al. [41]; Dhanjal et al. [42]). Aging is unique for everyone; therefore, elder care must be person-centered. Individuals are bio-psychosocial beings operating dynamically within an ever-changing society. Hence, interventions for older persons should not only be individualized but also family-focused, culturally acceptable, and provided in nonrestrictive, age-friendly environments that promote autonomy, dignity, and healthy aging without "biomedicalization" of old age (WHO [10]; Jonsson [43]).

Providing comprehensive care based on the needs of the individual in a qualitative, coordinated, efficient, safe, affordable, and sustainable manner is what will ensure a better quality of life for older persons (WHO, [24, 11, 44]). Eldercare needs are varied and depend on the individual, functional ability, and society, and could range from physical, emotional, psychological, social, economic, spiritual, and environmental (Touhy and Jett, [26]). Senior citizens who enjoy healthy aging would have the physical ability and mental and cognitive alertness to serve in a variety of ways as elder statesmen, leaders, mentors, coaches, managers, and teachers, passing on valuable knowledge, skills, and experiences to the younger generation. Using their expertise, they could promote societal growth and socio-economic development. This, however, could only happen if they enjoy a measure of good health and functional ability that would enable them to do the things they desire and enjoy doing. The challenges would arise if no socio-economic policies and appropriate planning have been put in place to respond to the aging trend through the provision of lifelong health promotion, health maintenance, and disease prevention services and programs (Advanced Home Health Care, [45]). Adverse circumstances could also occur if integrated ways of managing chronic ailments and providing social care for older persons in need are not put in place. The same would be the case if agedcare is not cost-effective, affordable, culturally acceptable, and sustainable (WHO, [1]; Crawford, Stoye, and Zaranko, [46]). Aging-related challenges that could occur range from elder abuse and neglect, unmet health and social care needs, overwhelming of the acute care sector, social hospitalization, unhealthy aging, poor quality of life among older persons, and poor economic development. The above principles should form part of the discourse by developing nations charting a way forward for a suitable, LTC system that would promote the wellbeing of their older persons. LTC of elders should be part of the national economic strategic plan and should take a life course approach such that no one is left out. It should not be based on humanitarian grounds or out of sympathy.

In the United Nations Principles for Older Persons, adopted by the General Assembly Resolution 46 of 1991 and the General Assembly Resolution 37/51 of 1982, key issues concerning older persons, which were highlighted to be addressed in a systematic manner, were: independence, participation, health and social care, aging with self-fulfillment, and dignity. Building on and referring to other international policies, plans, covenants, and conventions, the UN called on all member nations to ensure appropriate policies, structures, and strategies are put in place to provide an enabling environment for older persons to enjoy healthy aging, better quality of life, care, and protection in order to thrive and continue benefiting and contributing to the society which they have worked so hard to build as young people and adults (UN General Assembly Resolution [47]; 1982 [48]). The First World Assembly on Ageing focused on strengthening the capacities of countries to address issues related to aging such as research, data, education and training, and sectors that have to do with health and nutrition, housing, environment, income security, and welfare (United Nations [48]). Interestingly, the Second World Assembly on aging built on and expanded the plan of the first. The focus was on ensuring older persons are supported to remain active and participate in national development, "advancing health till old age," and promoting an "age-friendly environment" (United Nations [49]).

The UN Decade of Healthy Ageing (2021–2030), aimed at improving health equity and the lives of older persons, their families, and communities through a collaborative and multisectoral approach, has reechoed the above facts. The key messages from the various assemblies on aging and international plans were summarized by the WHO under the call to action, which is very clear:

> *changing how we think, feel and act towards age and ageism; developing communities in ways that foster the abilities of older people; delivering person-centred integrated care and primary health services responsive to older people; and providing older people who need it with access to quality long-term care*
> (WHO [10])

The focus, therefore, for developing and underdeveloped nations, and indeed the whole world, should be the promotion of functional abilities of seniors, integrating health and social care with the primary healthcare system serving as a hub or focal point for the provision of flexible, acceptable, quality, sustainable agedcare close to where older persons live. Ensuring that the issues of cost and access are addressed so that all elders who need LTC receive it. The public health issue of concern, according to the WHO [11], is that at least 75% of older adults will require assistance or LTC for basic daily activities at some point in their lives. Worldwide, around 142 million older adults, about 14% of the population across 42 countries, have unmet LTC needs (WHO [11]). This is the challenge that all nations must address, especially the developing and underdeveloped nations.

Agedcare or LTC, at its inception, has always been considered the responsibility of the family. Humanitarian agencies only stepped in to help after realized how overwhelming the situation was. Subsequently, the government responded by setting up a formal framework for agedcare. Hospitals have traditionally been designed for acute care; however, as older persons were admitted for acute and sometimes chronic diseases, they often ended up staying longer due to their multiple noncommunicable or long-term ailments, limitations, disabilities, and associated LTC needs. Some studies revealed that caring for older persons with chronic illnesses in hospitals was costly and not a sustainable model (Akingunola et al. [16]; Barajas-Nava et al. [50]; Flaherty et al. [51]). These studies indicated that complications arising from prolonged hospitalization would further increase the cost of care in hospitals. This model was, at times, inconvenient for older persons and their care givers. The LTC needs outside the traditional healthcare services, which hospitals were designed for, were not met, leading to dissatisfaction. This situation also often resulted in the blocking of bed spaces intended for acute care. The outcomes for clients were not better; rather, some adverse effects were observed, including hospital-acquired infections, stiffness of the joints resulting in poor mobility, and the absence of comprehensive agedcare services due to the fast pace of activities in acute care settings, among others (WHO [15]; Denham [52]). Based on these findings, recommendations were made for older persons with chronic conditions to be cared for in specialized or designated hospitals with trained physicians, nurses, and personal care support workers to deliver comprehensive management, palliative care, health and social care, and support services (Flaherty et al. [51]). It was against this background that the design of home and community-based LTC started receiving attention. Most developed countries that responded to the challenges of providing LTC to older persons are still tackling major issues in the sector to promote inclusivity and sustainability. These include issues of cost, choice, human resources, and quality, as seen in the United Kingdom and the United States of America (Crawford et al. [46]; State of New Jersey Department of Banking and Finance [53]). The studies mentioned above did not suggest that home or community care would be outrightly cheaper, but they highlighted several points. First, if chronic diseases are identified early and treatment is instituted in a timely manner, complications could be reduced, thereby saving treatment costs. Secondly, when health promotion and disease prevention strategies are adopted early enough by older persons, most chronic ailments could be avoided. When a chronic ailment has been diagnosed and treatment started, appropriate palliative care and education on self-care can be instituted without frequent recourse to hospitals. To implement these strategies, the home-community-primary healthcare system becomes the most viable option.

2.2 Moving LTC into homes and communities in developing and underdeveloped nations

There is no one-size-fits-all LTC system for older persons. LTC models vary and depend largely on the functional ability of the individual needing care, the environment, and available resources. These could include residential care facilities, respite care, nursing homes, assisted living arrangements, and hospital-based care. Models that utilize home, community, and primary healthcare systems for health and social care, appropriately linked to secondary and tertiary hospitals for acute care when necessary, have been advocated based on identified benefits over hospital-based long-term or purely residential care facilities (WHO [15, 11]). Homecare involves the provision of healthcare and social care services or medical supplies directly to individuals in their residences in the community (National Clinical Homecare Association [54]). Community-based LTC provides a critical link between the home and community in the continuum of integrated LTC care. Community-based services include respite care, recreation, social networking, information dissemination, training and education, health check-ups and screening, as well as the provision of consumables. The primary healthcare system could play an important role as the formal care hub through which agedcare activities around the home and community revolve, serving as the first entry point for primary agedcare, provision of consumables, appliances, support services, training and education, check-ups and screening, as well as assessment. It can provide support for community centers and formal and informal carers. An integrated LTC system that is provided at home and in the community with formal care givers, professional health and agedcare personnel, supported by trained informal carers, has been advocated and successfully implemented by many developed nations and some emerging economies. Examples include Sweden, which focuses on the training and support of informal care givers, and countries like Australia, Japan, the UK, and the USA, which provide home and community agedcare services supported by the government, to name a few.

The basic question that should be answered is: who should decide on the type of LTC model to use? The older persons themselves would be the forthright answer for many, and rightly so, if the individual has the capacity to do so. If not, recourse to the advanced care directive would provide the necessary guidance. Considerations such as the choice of the elders themselves and their families, society, culture, environment, and availability of a home, among others, usually determine the option. The community, social networks available, amenities in the home, and accessibility to home-based care packages, among other factors, are issues that older persons may likely consider in making a choice, as indicated in **Figure 3** below by Mah et al. [55].

In this work, an attempt will be made to highlight the LTC models of choice preferred by elders across various developing and a few developed countries.

Therefore, for home and community agedcare services to succeed, they must be properly organized and coordinated, and the required personnel must be available. This will ensure that nurses, personal care support workers, geriatricians or community physicians, and other therapists are readily available to provide health and social care, adequate nutrition, and physical and emotional support to elders in their familiar environment (Bakerjian [56]).

2.3 Efforts in some emerging and developing economies toward modifying LTC

Some emerging economies as China and Brazil have shown that a more grassroot centered approach that addresses LTC from the home, community, and primary healthcare approach holds a lot of advantages in terms of cost, flexibility, proximity to the older persons and their family as well as acceptability. The Brazil's health and social care systems are organized and coordinated across the local government authorities and implemented using the structures of the primary healthcare system to effectively reach older persons with LTC (Lloyd-Sherlock, Giacomin and Sempé [57], Aredes et al. [58]. China, though overwhelmed initially rose to the occasion by developing community based agedcare system to provide lifelong education and comprehensive LTC for older persons using community-based structures and resources (Yue et al. [59]).

For some developing countries in Africa, significant changes have occurred, and more are expected in the future if the tempo is sustained. South Africa, Seychelles, and Mauritius have developed long-term systems with social security that are ongoing. These countries have made progress in developing LTC systems, including rights-based legal frameworks, government-funded services, and monitoring mechanisms. However, challenges such as unmet demand, financial sustainability, and workforce shortages persist. Seychelles has the highest life expectancy in Africa and the highest percentage of elders in the population in Africa, courtesy of its sound eldercare social support system. Some forms of agedcare in Kenya and Ghana are also being implemented. Kenya's private nursing agencies and South Africa's Rand Aid are models of LTC that integrate family involvement, person-centered care, caregiver training, and health service linkages, but they remain limited in scale and accessibility. Nigeria, with the largest population in Africa of about 220 million and an absolute number of seniors aged 60 years and above of over 10 million (4%), just started about four years ago laying the foundational structures for the care of older persons following the establishment of the National Senior Citizen Centre (NSCC) [71] – an agency of the Federal Government – in May, 2021. Under the auspices of the NSCC, some teaching hospitals with geriatric departments have been supported to start training geriatric social support workers, personal support workers, and caregivers. Efforts are under way toward the construction of senior centers for community-based eldercare services in the six geopolitical regions and then in all state capitals. This is intended to catalyze the construction of similar centers in the 774 local government authorities and subsequently in every community through a public-private partnership. This will be a quantum leap forward if achieved (National Senior Citizen Centre [60]).

The Nursing and Midwifery Council of Nigeria (NMCN) has developed a very comprehensive curriculum in gerontology nursing for the specialty education of registered nurses as gerontology nurses. In early 2024, the NMCN granted accreditation to the first Gerontology Nursing Programme at the University of Benin Teaching Hospital, Benin City, Edo State, Nigeria. This is not only the first of its kind in Nigeria but also in Africa, south of the Sahara, excluding South Africa. Curricula for Post graduate studies in Gerontology Nursing are also ready for universities with the capacity to take them up (NMCN [61]).

2.4 Considerations for moving LTC from hospital to home, community, and primary healthcare settings: the way forward

Having set the above background, the model of LTC be provided for older persons whether they are living with or without disabilities cannot be the same across any country. What should concern policy makers, health planners and managers as well as health and agedcare professionals is the model of care that is acceptable, accessible, that would guarantee the wellbeing, satisfaction, better quality of life, dignity and independence of older persons. The basic issues that must be addressed to achieve this include: development of appropriate comprehensive eldercare policy backed up by legislation, designing of integrated LTC of system, utilization of data, capacity development- training of professionals, formal and informal caregivers, reactivation of the primary healthcare system and incorporation of eldercare services and healthy ageing programs.

Eldercare policy framework should be linked with the health policy and should operate within already existing systems and structures to avoid duplication or redundancy. Issues to be addressed should be comprehensive, including health and social care, elder abuse redress mechanisms, home modification and living arrangements, training and flexible engagement, age-friendly environments, sustainable financing models, support for informal care givers, coordination, governance issues, data utilization, monitoring, and evaluation, among others, as highlighted in **Figure 4**.

The aging curve, though not universal, is associated with peculiar needs that must be addressed in a comprehensive and well-coordinated manner if elders are to live longer, remain active, and functional, and contribute their wealth of experience and knowledge to building society. Challenges such as declining functional ability, multimorbidity, and comorbidities could either be prevented or properly managed with robust, well-coordinated, and regulated health and agedcare systems that focus on disease prevention and health promotion, as well as integrate care and social support from the home to community centers through to primary healthcare facilities and hospitals when necessary. Posthospital care could be provided at respite centers, residential care facilities, or nursing homes when required. The older person can also be discharged directly to their homes if home-based and community-based care services are optimal, resulting in the maintenance of social connectivity with family and friends, reduced chances of loneliness, healthy aging and a longer life span. An integrated continuum of LTC should be the direction to pursue (WHO, [23]). Integrated care for older persons has been the globally encouraged approach because of its numerous benefits. However, integrated LTC for older persons cannot be complete without the home and community structures. The

Integrated Care for Older People (ICOPE) approach is the provision of a continuum of health and social care services required by older persons in a coordinated and nonfragmented manner through a range of appropriate models in a flexible and person-centered way (WHO [34]; Halter et al. [62]). The care could be provided at home, at the community level, at the primary healthcare level, in respite care, or in residential care, if necessary, as indicated many years ago, as shown in **Figure 5**.

Data holds a prime place in the planning and implementation of LTC. The number, gender, distribution, and age ranges of older persons, their respective locations, living arrangements, and available support are just some of the data that would be very useful for the central government, states, and local government authorities. Utilizing data for planning, implementation, and monitoring would contribute to success.

Education and continuous training of all personnel required for the provision of agedcare or LTC is a necessity. It does appear that many elders in developing nations receive care from informal caregivers. Therefore, training informal caregivers and supporting them with some allowances from the government would be a very innovative approach to cutting costs while improving the quality of home- and community-based LTC care. There can be no LTC without human resources.

The primary healthcare system in most developing nations is weak, with the primary healthcare system lacking requisite infrastructure, personnel, equipment, and services (Chizoba et al. [63], Udontre et al. [64]). In some studies conducted in Oyo State, Nigeria, from 2021 to 2023, using six local government areas to determine the quality of life of older persons in these counties as well as the responsiveness of the primary healthcare system to the healthcare and social support needs of older persons, it was found that only 2 out of the 12 primary healthcare centers had designated monthly clinic days for services and programs targeted at older persons. In a quasi-experimental study involving 468 elders aged 50 years and over, at least two health education sessions were conducted for elders brought together in the 12 primary healthcare centers in the 6 local government areas. The focus was on physical exercise, healthy nutrition, avoidance of harmful habits such as alcohol abuse, smoking, taking unprescribed medicines and local products, adequate sleep, recreation, and regular medical check-ups. Postintervention assessment after a period of six months indicated improvement in healthy habits (Udontre et al. [76]). Most of the older persons expressed willingness to attend the clinics in the primary healthcare centers if such services were available, noting that they previously lacked knowledge and information on health necessary for their self-care and wellbeing (Udontre et al.[65]). For LTC to be effective, the PHC structures must be made functional to serve as the first point of care and services after the home and to provide linkage between the home and community.

3. Models and conceptual frameworks that support transitioning LTC to home, community, and primary healthcare settings

There are numerous models and conceptual frameworks that support the effectiveness, efficiency, safety, sustainability, and suitability of home- and community-based LTC for older persons. Most of them support comprehensive eldercare and the integration of care across acute, subacute, and LTC settings along the life course in age-friendly and familiar environments.

The elements indicated in **Figure 1** highlight the multifaceted nature of factors contributing to healthy aging, better quality of life, and longevity, which must be addressed by a responsive eldercare system. The home, community, and primary

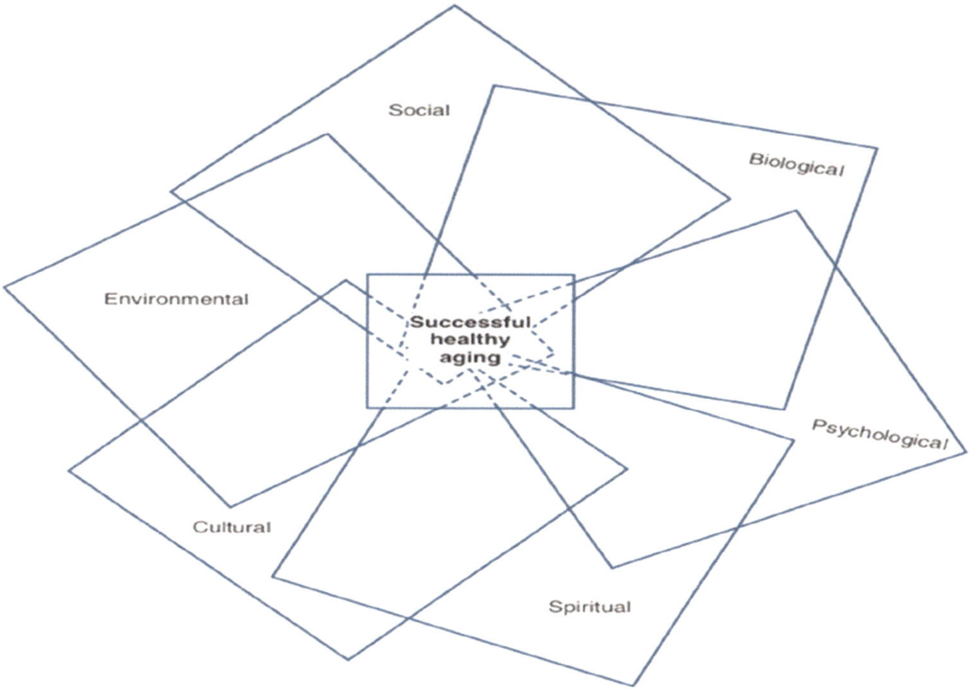

Figure 1.
Elements of healthy aging as developed by Patricia Hess (Touhy and Jett, [26]).

healthcare settings provide an environment that supports comprehensive agedcare services.

As indicated in **Figure 2**, several factors influence utilization of home care by elders based on the location, socio-cultural and environmental circumstances.

The innovative community-based eldercare system shown in **Figure 3** demonstrates how digital literacy, health promotion activities, culturally acceptable social engagement, health screening, treatment, and utilization of ICT can be utilized to promote healthy aging in China. It is a model that could be studied, adapted, and used by developing countries based on their socio-economic circumstances. Health education, health screening, and behavioral interventions are key modalities for positively influencing knowledge, attitudes, habits, and practices in favor of healthy aging and wellness among older persons.

The policy framework in **Figure 4** indicates that, for home and community-based care to be successful, the government must support it with appropriate policy and legislation. Consideration must be given to the governance structure, funding, human resources, and sustainability.

Figures 5 and **6** show that the integrated LTC model has been promoted over a long period. Halter et al. [62] wrote on it in 2016 indicating that homecare, acute care, subacute and LTC should be properly integrated to avoid segmentation and to ensure continuity of LTC and balance in the use of each component. In 2021, the WHO came up with the concept of integrated continuum of LTC. The basic components are similar with that of **Figure 5**, with some additional elements, showing that this model supports the principles of equity, accessibility, affordability, human dignity, and person centeredness.

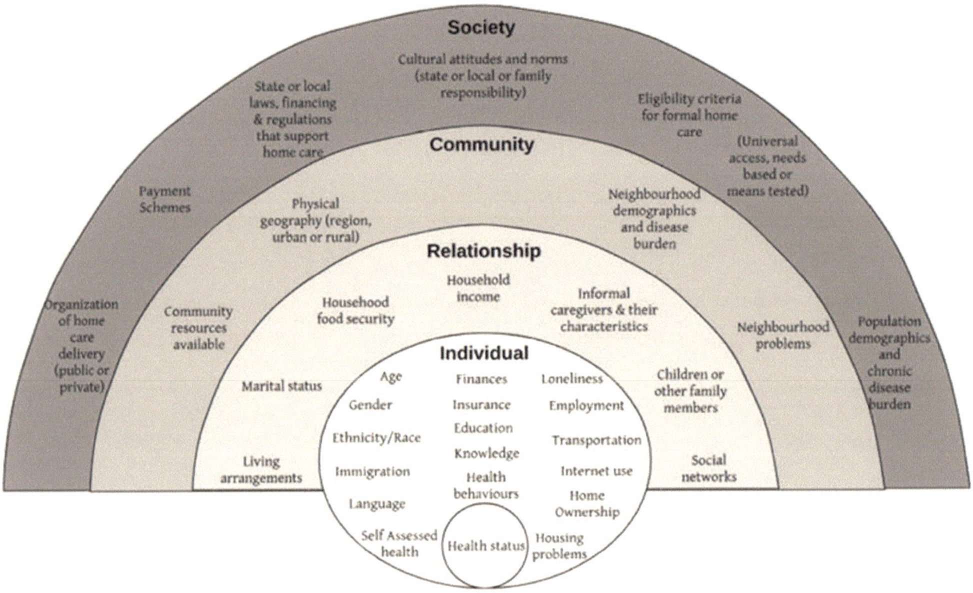

Figure 2.
Socio-ecological framework model indicating factors that influence the utilization of homecare services by older persons (Mah et al. [55]).

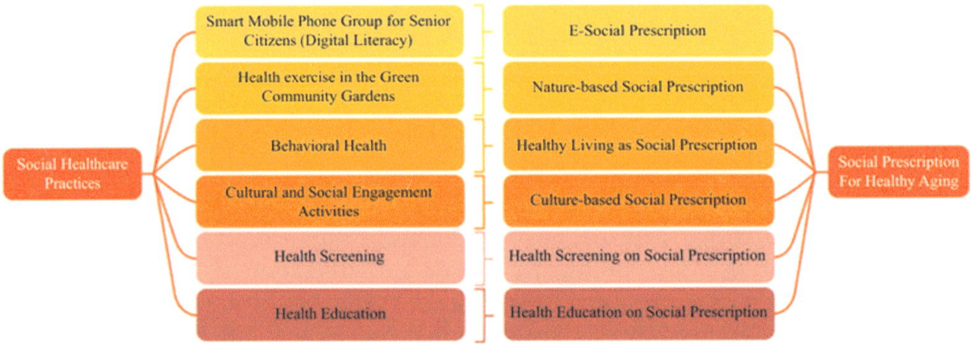

Figure 3.
An example of community-based social healthcare practices in China for healthy aging (Menhaset al. [66]).

4. Presentation and analysis of key findings from some studies in developing nations indicating older persons LTC preferences

Aging in place is the preference across many developing nations, as evidenced by the widespread choice of home- and community-based care by older persons, as shown in **Table 1** above. In the African setting and most Asian countries, residential care for older persons is not generally a welcome idea because it involves removing the older person from their home, relatives, neighbors and familiar surroundings. Home and family care are consistently preferred by older persons in Africa due to cultural norms of filial piety, dignity, and emotional support. This preference was observed in studies conducted in

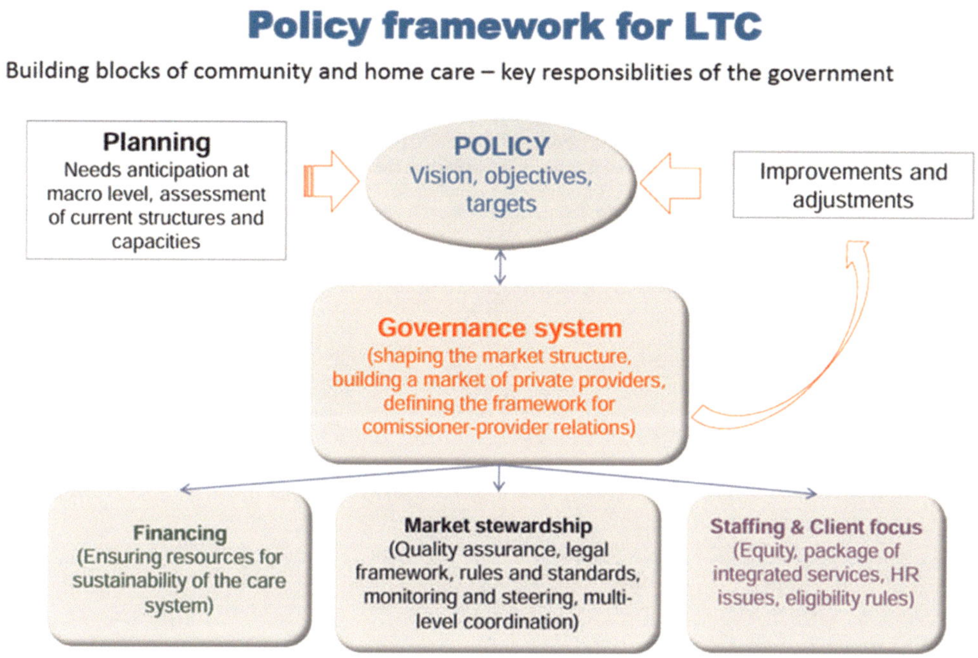

Figure 4.
Policy framework for the implementation of long-term care (O'Keefe [67]).

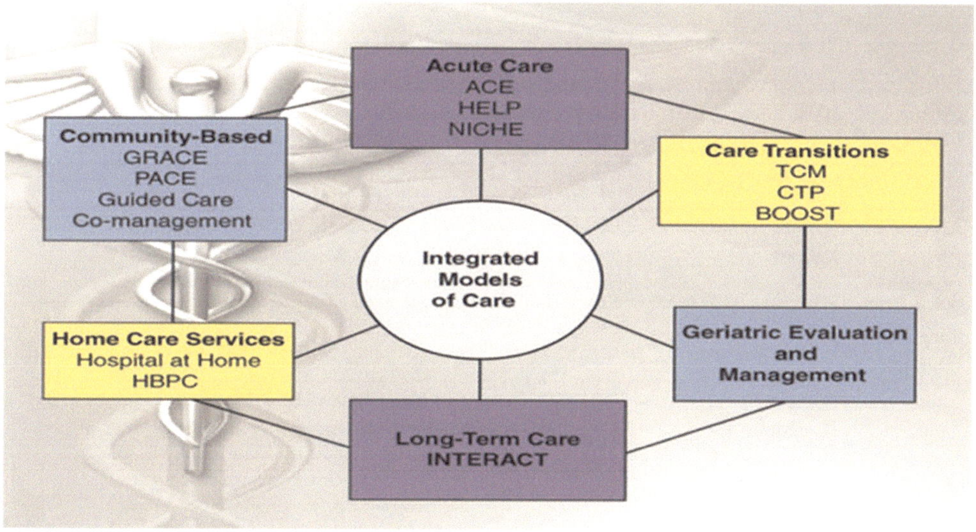

Figure 5.
Integrated model of care for older persons (source: Halter et al. [62]).

Nigeria, Kenya, South Africa, China, and Vietnam (Cadmus et al. [22]; Mussie et al. [68]). Some studies in three developed economies – conducted in the USA, UK, and Japan – indicated that a large percentage of elders preferred home and community-based care. In a US study of 2,826 adults aged 50 years and above, 77% of adults preferred

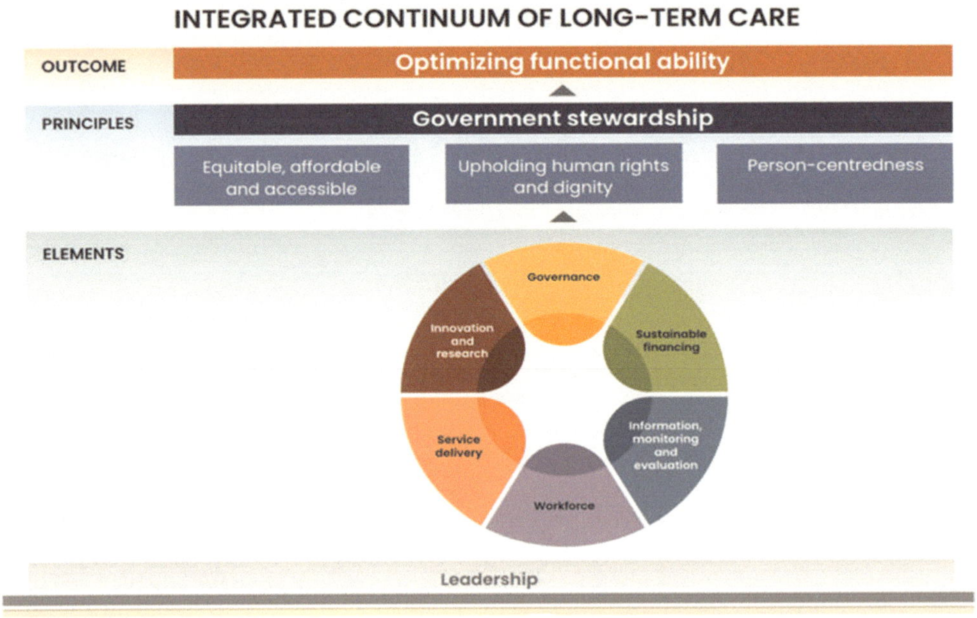

Figure 6.
Framework for achieving an integrated continuum of long-term care (World Health Organization [11]).

Country/ region	Year of study	Sample	Key finding (preferences)	Sources
Nigeria (Oyo State)	2023	1,180 community-dwelling older persons (aged 60 years and over)	Majority preferred to receive long-term care at home with family support; institutional care was the least preferred.	[22]
Eastern Africa (Ethiopia, Kenya, Tanzania, Uganda)	2022 (scoping review)	Review of 45 studies on older persons' care	Found family and home-based care were the dominant and culturally accepted models; institutional care was viewed as abandonment.	[68]
China	Chinese Longitudinal Healthy Longevity Study, 2018		Majority of the elders and their families reported a preference for home-based care. Community hospitals and primary health centers are utilized due to a shortage of formal caregivers.	[69]
China (Jiangsu Province)	2024 Cross sectional survey	870 older persons	60.11% preferred home-based care, while 13% preferred residential care	[70]

Country/ region	Year of study	Sample	Key finding (preferences)	Sources
Vietnam	Data of Vietnam Aging Survey	4,002 elders aged 50 years and above, out of which 2,798 were 60 years and above were surveyed across 12 provinces in 6 zones.	Care of older persons is mainly provided by family members and relatives: 42.44% by spouses, 43.13% by daughters, 37.04% by sons, 34.67% by daughters-in-law, and 19.38% by granddaughters.	[71]
Latin America and the Caribbeans	Analysis and report by experts from the Pan-American Health Organization, the United Nations, and the Inter-American System	Data on long-term care and services in the Latin America and Caribbean subregion indicates that Argentina, Brazil, Uruguay, and Chile have some innovative public and social care programs.	Many Latin American and Caribbean countries lack an LTC system for dependent older people regulated by a national policy. Care is mainly home-based. Argentina: 77% of elderly individuals are cared for by family members, while 3.4% are cared for by specialized care workers. Uruguay: 82% of care is provided by unpaid care givers, and 58.9% is provided by family members. Brazil: 35.1% of elders aged 50 years and above who need LTC receive it from family (94.1%), 72.1% of whom are females.	Pan [72]

Table 1.
Presentation and analysis of key findings from various studies in developing nations indicating older persons' LTC preferences.

home-based care. Japan has shifted its focus from providing on LTC in large geriatric centers to supporting older adults to age in place whenever possible (AARP [73]; Age UK [74]; Ukawa et al. [75]). Apart from homecare, community services also strengthen aging in place and are preferred. These services have been linked to improved wellbeing when available. In countries deeply entrenched in the cultural belief that family members should care for their older relatives out of the philosophy of filial piety and respect, most family members have little or no capacity in terms of knowledge, skills, and economic power (Kyeong et al. [76]). Therefore, there is a need to train more formal care givers as well as informal care givers to improve the quality of care that elders receive in home and community-based care settings.

5. Summary

History is there to teach us about the past, so we can navigate the future with wisdom without repeating previous mistakes. In the early days of LTC, older persons were left to the care of families and charitable agencies. Later, various residential care facilities were developed for the long-term care of older persons, including nursing homes, assisted living, and hospice. After a series of evaluations and reviews, home- and community-based care has been adopted by many nations because of its numerous benefits, especially supporting aging in place, proximity, acceptability, accessibility, and affordability.

The range and degree of LTC required for various older people would vary depending on their environment, functional ability and unique physical, emotional, psychological, and cognitive abilities as well as the networks available. The basic issues such as a supportive environment, education on adequate nutrition, leisure and entertainment, adequate sleep, adherence to treatment regimen where applicable, promotion of healthy lifestyle and habits, education on self-care could be achieved at home, community and primary healthcare settings with little cost on the part of the service providers and the recipients of care. Other services such as medical/health checks, palliative care, care of activities of daily living can be incorporated, coordinated and provided at affordable rates at the home-community-primary healthcare settings. A public health system with interventions focused on disease prevention and health promotion, age friendly environment, healthy nutrition, leading of active life as well as lifestyle modifications should be designed, and the primary healthcare facilities should be used as a hub and focal point for reaching out to older adults and their families and homes. Capacity development and training of personnel such as personal support workers, carers, geriatric social workers, gerontologists, gerontology nurses, geriatricians, occupational or recreational therapists, among others must be pursued vigorously because there would be no care without the personnel with the right competencies. Training and remuneration of informal carers as done in Sweden, one of the foremost countries to experience ageing, is a lesson for developing nations. If informal caregivers are trained and supported with some allowances and placement on flexible employment, then a huge gap in human resource would be filled since most LTC in developing countries take place at home. The development of appropriate comprehensive eldercare policy backed up by legislation, the design and implantation of integrated LTC system, utilization of data, capacity development- training of professionals, formal and informal caregivers, reactivation of the primary healthcare system with incorporation of eldercare services and healthy ageing programs are viable steps to be taken in developing nations going forward.

6. Conclusion

The available body of evidence supports the fact that older persons in most developing nations depend on family members for LTC. However, many adult children have left their homes for foreign countries or urban cities due to push and pull factors and are not available to provide care. Young women, who were traditionally family caregivers, are now taking up full-time employment, and community structures have disintegrated due to the absence of extended family systems. Informal caregivers are neither trained nor supported, the formal regulated agedcare system is still at a rudimentary stage, and the primary health system, which is supposed to be the first gate way to care, is dysfunctional and under-resourced. Under these circumstances, hospitals, which are meant to be acute care center have become hubs for both acute and chronic ailments. Older persons often spend months in hospitals, some meeting the end of their lives surrounded by nurses and doctors in uniforms rather than family members. There are no parting words to the children left behind at death because they are not present in the first place. This scenario must change in developing nations if older persons in need of LTC are to enjoy better quality of life, independence, dignity, autonomy, and appropriate social support until the very end of life. Home- and community-based LTC would enhance the involvement of family and friends in care promote independence, autonomy, and comfort due to the maintenance of attachment to a familiar environment. Home- and community-based care also fosters connectivity with loved ones. The comfort of one's home can promote wellbeing, and it is cheaper and more sustainable than LTC in residential care facilities and hospitals. In providing care for older persons, the aim should be to continue adding good health to long life by delivering quality, accessible, acceptable, affordable, integrated, and sustainable LTC that promotes healthy aging and a better quality of life. Governments in developing nations should be proactive in designing and implementing appropriate eldercare policies backed by legislation and funding. Reactivating the primary healthcare system and integrating eldercare services into homes and community centers are essential steps to be taken. Capacity development for formal care providers and training and support for informal caregivers are necessities. The work has been laid out for developing and underdeveloped nations, courtesy of gerontogrowth and population aging and the time to act is now.

Author details

Emmanuel Edet Udontre[1,2,3,4,5,6]

1 Nursing, University of Nigeria, Enugu, Nigeria

2 Applied Gerontology, Flinders University, Adelaide, Australia

3 Diploma in Strategic Leadership and Management, MSBM, UK

4 Community/Public Health Nursing, LAUTECH, Nigeria

5 RN, FWAPCNM – Head of Department, Education, Nursing, and Midwifery Council of Nigeria, Nigeria

6 Part-Time Lecturer, Gerontology Nursing Programa, University of Benin Teaching Hospital, Benin City, Nigeria

*Address all correspondence to: emmanueludontre@gmail.com

References

[1] World Health Organization. Ageing: Global Population. Geneva. 2025. Available from: https://www.who.int/news-room/questions-and-answers/item/population-ageing [Accessed: 2025-March-20]

[2] United Nations Department of Economic and Social Affairs. World Population Prospects 2024. Summary of Results, United Nations: New York. 2024. Available from: https://www.un.org/development/desa/pd/sites/www.un.org.development.desa.pd/files/undesa_pd_2024_wpp_2024_advance_unedited_0.pdf [Accessed: 2025-October-02]

[3] Cook IG, Halsall J. Aging in Comparative Perspective: Processes and Policies. Vol. **11**. Article 8: Springer Science & Business Media; 2011 949781461419785. https://scholar.google.com.au/scholar?hl=en&q=Cook+and+Halsall++%282012%29+Aging+in+Comparative+Perspective+Processes+and+policies&btnG=&as_sdt=1%2C5&as_sdtp= DOI: 10.1007/978-1-4614-1978-5 [Accessed: 2025-June-21]

[4] National Research Council (US) Panel on a Research Agenda and New Data for an Aging World. Preparing for an Aging World: The Case for Cross-National Research. Vol. **2**. Washington (DC): National Academies Press (US); 2001. Our Aging World: Available from: https://www.ncbi.nlm.nih.gov/books/NBK98375 [Accessed: 2025-July-03]

[5] United Nations Department of Economic and Social Affairs. Leaving No One Behind in An Ageing World.World Social Report 2023. https://www.un.org/development/desa/dspd/wp-content/uploads/sites/22/2023/01/2023wsr-chapter1-.pdf [Accessed: 2025-May-11] (New York USA: United Nations Department of Economic and Social Affairs)

[6] Taylor P, Powell P. The Global South:The case of population aging in Africa and Asia. World Scientific News. 2015;(6):89–99. https://worldscientific.com [Accessed: 2025-September-30]

[7] United Nations Department of Economic and Social Affairs, Population Division. World Population Ageing 2013. ST/ESA/SER.A/348. New York: United Nations; 2013. Available from: https://www.un.org/en/development/desa/population/publications/pdf/ageing/WorldPopulationAgeing2013.pdf [Accessed: 2025-May-23]

[8] Francisco A. Gerontogrowth Vs. Population Ageing: Why Does This Differentiation Matters? 21st International Association of Gerontology and Geriatrics World Congress. San Fransico: Instituto du Escudos Social e Economicus (IESE); 2017

[9] Francisco A. 'Gerontogrowth' and Population Ageing in Africa and the Global Age Watch Index. Mozambique: Institute for Social and Economic Studies (IESE), Economic Faculty of the Eduardo Mondlane University; 2016

[10] World Health Organization. Ageing and Health. Key Facts. 2024. https://www.who.int/news-room/fact-sheets/detail/ageing-and-health [Accessed: 2025-June-02]

[11] World Health Organization. Framework for countries to achieve an integrated continuum of long-term care. 2021. Geneva: WHO.CCBY-NC-SA3.

0IGO, chrome-extension://efaidnbmnn nibpcajpcglclefindmkaj/https://iris.who.int/bitstream/handle/10665/349911/9789240038844-eng.pdf? [Accessed: 2025-June-02]

[12] World Bank Group. Silver Opportunity: Case Studies-Long-Term Care for Aging Populations in Africa: Current Landscape, Key Challenges, and Policy Considerations. n d. Available from: https://documents1.worldbank.org/curated/ [Accessed: 2025-June-02]

[13] World Health Organization. Towards Long-term care systems in sub-Saharan Africa. 2017.WHO Series on Long-term Care on Healthy Ageing. Available from: https://www.who.int/publications/i/item/9789241513388 [Accessed: 2025-July-20]

[14] United Nations, Economic and Social Commission for Asia and the Pacific (ESCAP).Asia-Pacific Report on Population Ageing 2022: Trends, Policies and Good Practices regarding Older Persons and Population Ageing. 2022. ST/ESCAP/3041 [Accessed: 2025-October-30]

[15] World Health Organization.Long-term Care for Older People-package for Universal Health Coverage. Geneva: WHO.CCBY-NC-SA3.0 IGO; 2024. https://iris.who.int/ [Accessed: 2025-August-02]

[16] Akingunola O, Sogunle T, Kareem Y, Egua L. Health-care utilisation among elderly people with chronic medical conditions in a Secondary Health-Care Center, Southwestern Nigeria. Nigerian Journal of Medicine. 2024;**33**:73–79. DOI: 10.4103/NJM.NJM_60_24 [Accessed: 2025-June-23]

[17] Jeyasingam N, McLean L, Mitchell L, Wand AP. Attitudes to ageing amongst health care professionals: A qualitative systematic review. European Geriatric Medicine. 2023;**14**(5):889–908. DOI: 10.1007/s41999-023-00841-7

[18] Australian Government Department of Health, Disability and Ageing. Commonwealth Home Support Program. 2025. Available from: https://www.health.gov.au/our-work/chsp?language=en [Accessed: 2025-October-25]

[19] Abdi S, Spann A, Borilovic J, de Witte L, Hawley M. Understanding the care and support needs of older people: A scoping review and categorisation using the WHO international classification of functioning, disability and health framework (ICF). BMC Geriatrics. 2019;**19**(1):195. DOI: 10.1186/s12877-019-1189-9 [Accessed: 2025-May-30]

[20] United Nations Economic Commission for Europe Active Ageing Index United Nations Economic Commission for Europe. 2018. Available from: https://unece.org/population/active-ageing-index (Geneva) [Accessed: 2025-October-30]

[21] Thaver I. Ageing in developing countries: Who cares? 2025. Available from: https://apolitical.co/solution-articles/en/ageing-in-developing-countries-who-cares [Accessed: 2025-April-2]

[22] Cadmus EO, Adebusoye LA, Owoaje ET. Ageing in place or stuck in place: Preferred care setting for community-dwelling older persons in a low-resource country in Sub Saharan Africa. PLoS One. 2023;**18**(10): e0292939. DOI: 10.1371/journal.pone.0292939 [Accessed: 2025-July-29]

[23] World Health Organization. Integrated Continuum of Long-Term Care. 2025. Available from: https://www.who.int/teams/maternal-newborn-child-adolescent-health-and-ageing/ageing-and-health/integrated-continuum-of-long-term-care [Accessed: 2025-June-30]

[24] World Health Organization. Long-Term Care. 2022. Available from: https://www.who.int/europe/news-room/questions-and-answers/item/long-term-care [Accessed: 2025-June-22]

[25] Kar N. Care needs of older persons. Journal of Geriatric Care and Research. 2015;**2**:1–2 [Accessed: 2025-July-04]

[26] Touhy T, Jett K. Ebersole and Hess Gerontological Nursing and Healthy Aging, 4th Ed. 2014. Available from: https://repository.poltekkes-kaltim.ac.id/676/1/Ebersole [Accessed: 2025-September-30]

[27] Australian Institute of Health & Welfare. Older Australians. 2024. https://www.aihw.gov.au/reports/older-people/older-Australians/contents/aged-care [Accessed: 2025-May-28]

[28] Yue Z, Xiang N, Li H. The evolution trend of availability of China's community-based care services and its impact on the cognitive function of elderly people: 2008-2018. International Journal for Equity in Health. 2021;**20**:203. DOI: 10.1186/s12939-021-01544-w [Accessed: 2025-June-25]

[29] Ikegami N. Financing Long-term Care: Lessons from Japan. International Journal of Health Policy Management. 2019;**1.8**(8):462–466. DOI: 10.15171/ijhpm.2019.35

[30] Health and Social Care Services. Social Care 360: Expenditure. 2025. Available from: https://www.kingsfund.org.uk/insight-and-analysis/long-reads/social-care-360-expenditure [Accessed: 2025-June-22]

[31] Rosenwohl-Mack A, Schumacher K, Fang M-L, Fukuoka Y. A new conceptual model of experiences of aging in place in the United States: Results of a systematic review and meta-ethnography of qualitative studies. International Journal of Nursing Studies. 2020;**103**:1–35. DOI: 10.1016/j.ijnurstu.2019.103496 [Accessed: 2025-June-02]

[32] Graybill EM, McMeekin P, Wildman J. Can aging in place be cost effective? A systematic review. PLoS One. 2014;**9**(7):e102705. DOI: 10.1371/journal.pone.0102705

[33] World Health Organization. Integrated Continuum of Long-term care. 2025. Available from: https://www.who.int/teams/maternal-newborn-child-adolescent-health-and-ageing/ageing-and-health/integrated-continuum-of-long-term- care# [Accessed: 2025-July-29]

[34] World Health Organization. Integrated Care of Older Person Approach. 2025. Available from: https://www.who.int/teams/maternal-newborn-child-adolescent-health-and-ageing/ageing-and-health/integrated-care-for-older-people-icope [Accessed: 2025-August-02]

[35] Gibson K, Kingston A, McLellan E, Louise Robinson L, Brittain K. Successful ageing in later older age: A sociology of class and ageing in place. Social Science & Medicine. 2024;**358**(117258):117258. DOI: 10.1016/j.socscimed.2024.117258

[36] Kok L, Berden C, Sadiraj K. Costs and benefits of home care for the

elderly versus residential care: A comparison using propensity scores. European Journal of Health Economics. 2015; **16**(2):119–131. DOI: 10.1007/s10 198-013-0557- [Accessed: 2025-August-02]

[37] Amarya S, Singh K, Sabharwal M. Ageing process and physiological changes. In: D'Onofrio, Grazia, Greco, Antonio, D' Onofrio, SancarloGrazia, editors. Gerontology. London, UK: IntechOpen; 2018. p. 1–24. DOI: 10.5772/intechopen.76249 [Accessed: 2025-March-12]

[38] United Nations Department of Economic and Social Affairs World Economic Situation and Prospects 2024. Available from: https://www.un.org/development/desa/dpad/wp-content/uploads/sites=/45/WESP_2024_Web.pdf [Accessed: 2025-April-28]

[39] UNDP. Destination2030 Accelerating Progress on the Sustainable Development Goals. 2025. Available from: https://www.undp.org/ [Accessed: 2025-June-12]

[40] Abdi S, Spann A, Borilovic J, de Witte L, Hawley M. Understanding the care and support needs of older people: A scoping review and categorisation using the WHO international classification of functioning, disability and health framework (ICF). BMC Geriatrics. 2019;**19**(1):195. DOI: 10.118 6/s12877-019-1189-9 [Accessed: 2025-May-30]

[41] Haupt S, Niedrist T, Sourij H, Schwarzinger S, Moser O. The impact of exercise on telomere length, DNA methylation and metabolic footprints. Cells. 2022;**11**(1):153

[42] Dhanjal DS, Bhardwaj S, Sharma R, Bhardwaj K, Kumar D, Chopra C, Nepovimova E, Singh R, Kuca K. Plant fortification of the diet for Anti-ageing effects: A review. Nutrients. 2020;**12** (10):3008/10 https://pubmed.ncbi.nlm.nih.gov/33007945/. DOI: 10.3390/nu12103008 [Accessed: 2025-October-02]

[43] Jonsson AB. Medicalization of old age: Experiencing healthism and overdiagnosis in a Nordic Welfare state. Available from: https://www.tandfonline.com/doi/full/ DOI: 10.1080/01459740.2024.2349515 [Accessed: 2025-June-20]

[44] World Health Organization. Global Strategy and Action Plan on Ageing and Health. Geneva:World Health Organization; 2017. CCBY-NC-SA3.0 IGO [Accessed: 2025-April-03]

[45] Advanced Home Health Care. We Can All Benefit from Seniors Becoming Mentors. 2022. Available from: https://advanced-homehealthcare.com/we-can-all-benefit-from-seniors-becoming-mentors/ (Burlington, USA) [Accessed: 2025-May-20]

[46] Crawford R, Stoye G, Zaranko B. Long-term care spending and hospital use among the older population in England. Journal of Health Economics. 2021;**78**:102477. https://www.sciencedirect.com/science/article/pii/S016762962100062X DOI: 10.1016/j.jhealeco.2021.102477 [Accessed: 2025-October-01]

[47] United Nations. 1991 United Nations Principles for Older Persons. Available from: https://www.ohchr.org/sites/default/files/olderpersons.pdf (Geneva) [Accessed: 2025-June-02]

[48] United Nations. First World Assembly on Ageing. 1982. Available from: https://www.un.org/en/

conferences/ageing/vienna1982 [Accessed: 2025-August-02]

[49] United Nations. Second World Assembly on Ageing Adopts Madrid International Plan of Action and Political Declaration. 2002. Available from: https://www.ohchr.org/en/press-releases/2009/10/second-world-assembly-ageing-adopts-madrid-international-plan-action-and# [Accessed: 2025-May-27]

[50] Barajas-Nava LA, Garduño-Espinosa J, Mireles Dorantes JM, Medina-Campos R, García-Peña MC. Models of comprehensive care for older persons with chronic diseases: A systematic review with a focus on effectiveness. Biomedical Journal Open. 2022;**12**(8): e059606. DOI: 10.1136/bmjopen-2021-059606 [Accessed: 2025-April-02]

[51] Flaherty JH, Rodin MB, Morley JE. Changing Hospital Care for Older Adults: The case for Geriatric Hospitals in the United States. Gerontology and Geriatric Medicine. 2022;8. DOI: 10.1177/23337214221109005

[52] Denham M 23June. A Brief History of the Care of the ElderlyJournal of British Geriatric Society. 2016. https://www.bgs.org.uk/resources/a-brief-history-of-the-care-of-the-elderly (London, United Kingdom) [Accessed: 2025-October-20]

[53] State of New Jersey Department of Banking and Finance. What You Should Know About Long-Term Care. Office of the Insurance Ombudsman. 2011. New Jersey. Available from: https://www.nj.gov/dobi/ins_ombudsman/ltcguide.htm [Accessed: 2025-October-30]

[54] National Clinical Homecare Association. Domiciliary Care or Home Care. 2011. Available from: https://www.clinicalhomecare.org/

[55] Mah JC, Stevens SJ, Keefe JN, Rockwood K, Andrew MK. Social factors influencing utilization of home care in community-dwelling older adults: A scoping review. 2021. Available from: https://www.academia.edu/62349509/Social_factors_influencing_utilization_of_home_care_in_community_dwelling_older_adults_a_scoping_review?auto=download&email_work_card=download-paper

[56] Bakerjian D. Settings for Care for Older Adults. 2025. Available from: https://www.msdmanuals.com/home/older-people-s-health-issues/providingcare-to-older-adults/settings-for-care-for-older-adults [Accessed: 2025-July-29]

[57] Lloyd-Sherlock P, Giacomin K, Sempé L. The effects of an innovative integrated care intervention in Brazil on local health service use by dependent older people. BMC Health Services Research. 2022;**22**:176. DOI: 10.1186/s12913-022-07552- [Accessed: 2025-April-20]

[58] Aredes JS, Billings J, Giacomin KC, Lloyd-Sherlock P, Firmo JOA. Integrated care in the community: The case of the Programa Maior Cuidado (Older Adult Care Programme) in Belo Horizonte-Minas Gerais, BRA. International Journal of Integrated Care. 2021;**21**(2):28. DOI: 10.5334/ijic.5619 [Accessed: 2025-June-15]

[59] Yue Z, Xiang N, Li H, et al. The evolution trend of availability of China's community-based care services and its impact on the cognitive function of elderly people: 2008-2018. International Journal for Equity in Health. 2021; **20**:203 [Accessed: 2025-June-22]

[60] National Senior Citizens Centre (NSCC). One Community OneSenior Centre-NSCC Public Private Partnership Initiative. 2023. Available from: https://nscc.kingsley.net.ng/nscc-policy-guidelines/

[61] Nursing and Midwifery Council of Nigeria. Gerontology NursingCurriculum. Abuja, Nigeria: NMCN; 2024 [Accessed: 2025-May-01]

[62] Halter JB, Ouslander GJ, Studenenski S, High KP, Asthana S, Supiano MA, Ritchie C, Hazzard, Woolard NF. Hazzard's Geriatric Medicine andGerontology. 7th ed.2016

[63] Chizoba AF, Obioma AJ, Okika-Chizoba C, Olasunkanmi F, Dikas LF, Adogu P, Nickson S, Ukachukwu LK. HealthcareAccessibility and Affordability Measures among Older Persons in Rural Nigeria. Acta Scientific Medical Sciences. 2025;**9**(2) [Accessed: 2025-July-30]

[64] Udontre E, Olubiyi K, Oyadiran G, Ajibade B, Akinfolarin O. Effects ofeducational intervention on dietary pattern and nutrition intake among elders in Oyo State, Nigeria. International Journal of Science and Research (IJSR). 2023;**12**(12): 1481–1489. DOI: 10.21275/SR231213170245

[65] Udontre EE, Oyadiran GO, Obataze AJ. Assessment of the quality of life of older adults dwelling in a State in Nigeria andPotential interventions for improving their wellbeing. IOSR Journal of Nursing and HealthScience (IOSR-JNHS). 2025;**14**(1):08–18. DOI: 10.9790/1959-1401020818

[66] Menhas R, Yang L, Danish NR. Community-based social healthcare practicesin China for healthy aging: A social prescriptionperspective analysis. FrontierPublic Health. 2023;**11**:1252157. DOI: 10.3389/fpubh.2023.1252157

[67] O'Keefe P. Aged and Long-Term Care in the Developing World with a Focus on Asia.Sydney: World Bank; 2018. Available from: https://cepar.edu.au/sites/default/files/2-OKeefe.pdf [Accessed: 2025-October-03]

[68] Mussie KM, Setchell J, Elger BS, Kaba M, Memirie ST, Wangmo T. Care of OlderPersons in Eastern Africa: A Scoping Review ofEthical Issues. Frontiers in Public Health. 2022;**10**: 923097. DOI: 10.3389/fpubh.2022.923097

[69] Xiao F, Cao S, Xiao M, et al.(2023) Patterns of home care andcommunity support preferences among older adults with disabilities in China: A latent class analysis. BMC Geriatrics. (2023);**23**:117 [Accessed: 2025-June-23]

[70] Wang Y, Wang Y, Liu Y, et al. Factors influencing senior care and living preferences among older adults inJiangsu, China: A cross-sectional survey study. BMC Health Services Research. 2024;**24**:723 [Accessed: 2025-May-21]

[71] Giang LT, Nguyen NT, Pham TH, Manh P. Factors associatedwith receipt of informal care among the Vietnamese older persons: Evidence from a national survey. Frontiers in Public Health. 2023;**11**:1065851. https://pmc.ncbi.nlm.nih.gov/articles/PMC10031064/

[72] Pan-American Health Organization and Inter-American Development Bank. Long-termCare in Latin America and the Caribbean. Washington, D.C.: Pan American; 2023. DOI: 10.37774/9789275127155 [Accessed: 2025-Nov-01]

[73] American Association of RetiredPersons (AARP). Home and Community Preferences SurveyAmerican Association of Retired Persons. 2012. Available from: https://www.aarp.org/pri/topics/livable-communities/housing/2021-home-community-preferences/ [Accessed: 2025-January-12]

[74] Age UK. Briefing: Health and Care ofOlder People in England 2019Web Based Report. 2019. Available from: https://www.google.com/search?q=Age+UK%2C+2019 (England) [Accessed: 2025-May-10]

[75] Ukawa S, Kato Y, Lee Y, Ohara K, Mori K. FactorsInfluencing the Preferences for Homes as the Location for Long-term Care in Japanese Population. The Open Public Health Journal. 2022; https://openpublichealthjournal.com/VOLUME/16/ELOCATOR/e187494452303280/FULLTEXT/ DOI: 10.2174/18749445-v16-e230419-2022-178 [Accessed: 2025-May-01]

[76] Kyeong Y, Yu M, Tiemeier H, Bakermans-Kranenburg MJ, Setoh P. Filial PietyAcross Sociocultural Context and the Life Span. Current Directions in PsychologicalScience. 2025;**34**(3):163–170 [Accessed: 2025-July-17]

Chapter 8

Perspective Chapter: Juxtaposing the Courtesy Stigma of Mental Illness and Family Caregiver Role Strain

Keletwaetse Sakwape, Miriam M. Moagi, Wada Gaolaolwe and Gaotswake Patience Kovane

Abstract

Caregiving is a complex role requiring one to juggle multiple and often competing demands. Caregivers of individuals with mental illness face various challenges, such as meeting their loved ones' needs, managing their behaviour when they are not mentally stable, and dealing with feelings related to courtesy stigma associated with mental illness. While family caregivers are the main source of support for those with mental illness, the burden they endure can be overwhelming, especially since their strain is further intensified by the courtesy stigma these families encounter. Stigma results in social distancing and insufficient support, which has numerous adverse effects and can impact their quality of life, including financial strain, isolation due to limited time for leisure and socializing, shame, guilt, and more. Therefore, understanding how caregiver role strain intersects with the courtesy stigma of mental illness is vital to ensure that caregivers' unique needs, experiences, and challenges are recognized, enabling the development of more effective support services.

Keywords: family caregiver experiences, role strain, stigma, strategies for support, mental illness, caregiving

1. Introduction

A significant number of individuals with moderate to severe mental illness struggle to fulfil daily responsibilities due to impairments in cognitive and social skills, which greatly affect their quality of life [1]. Consequently, many suffering from mental illness depend on their family members for support, as these caregivers play an essential informal role in helping with everyday tasks. Nonetheless, this assistance can result in caregiver role strain (CRS). Caregiver strain, whether objective or subjective, has negative consequences for caregivers, especially those caring for family members with chronic psychiatric conditions requiring long-term care [2]. Subjective burden mainly pertains to carers' personal feelings developed during caregiving, whereas objective burden is characterized by events or activities linked to negative caregiving experiences [3]. Individuals with chronic mental illnesses like dementia and schizophrenia require continuous long-term support and care, and their caregivers tend to have the lowest quality of life [4]. Caregivers must juggle various roles and responsibilities while monitoring their loved ones' symptoms, which can negatively impact their health, quality of life, social connections, and finances. Caregivers of people with chronic mental illnesses such as schizophrenia often experience stress from continuous caregiving responsibilities, even during remission, as well as social exclusion by their communities [5]. Although the family remains a key support for individuals with mental illness, this challenge is worsened by social exclusion stemming from courtesy stigma linked to mental illness, which these families face [5–7].

While the family unit continues to be a fundamental source of strength for those with mental illness, the challenge is further intensified by the courtesy stigma associated with mental illness that these families encounter [7]. Stigma refers to a social phenomenon in which individuals perceived as having inferior qualities by the public face negative treatment and inequality [8–10]. Historically, stigma associated with mental illness has persisted throughout literature from medieval times to the present [8, 11]. This negative stereotyping, labelling, and discrimination not only targets people with mental illness (PMI) but also their family members due to their close association or courtesy stigma [7]. Courtesy stigma amplifies family CRS, eroding the families' social support networks.

2. Mental illness and stigma

2.1 Understanding mental illness

The understanding of the cause of mental illness has been the subject of contentious debate throughout history. Literature records divergent viewpoints, showing how people's perceptions of mental illness are influenced by time, culture, and civilization. Plato, in ancient Greece, was among the first to attempt to define mental illness, which was conceived as reason aided by temper and ruling over passion [12]. On the contrary, Hippocrates adopted a more physicalist approach, explaining mental phenomena and all aspects of human experience in terms of physical processes and entities. According to Hippocrates, different mental conditions are a result of various imbalances between types of "humours." However, in other regions of the world, mental illness was viewed as caused by supernatural forces, such as possession and sorcery, and treatment involved acts such as exorcism and purging. During that period, society widely held the belief that individuals grappling with psychiatric disorders or displaying unusual behaviours were under the malevolent influence of demons or were suffering divine retribution from God or the pantheon of gods for their transgressions. This pervasive outlook painted a vivid picture of torment and spiritual struggle, where the afflicted were often viewed not as victims of illness, but as pitiable souls trapped in a battle against supernatural forces or celestial judgment for their sins.

Pre-existing beliefs about the causes of mental illness influence a caregiver's perceptions of the caring experience and determine the kinds of attitudes they later adopt [7, 13]. This is because beliefs shape perceptions of encountered situations and guide actions taken, thereby affecting emotional outcomes. If the caregiver believes that mental illness in a relative is a result of punishment for their own misdeeds, they might feel guilt and stress, which can significantly worsen their role burden [7, 13, 14]. As a result, the caregiver, seeking to compensate for what they see as their misdeed, may become overly involved in the care – even in difficult situations where they need assistance. Caregivers holding such beliefs put much time and effort into caring for their family member with mental illness, trying to compensate for what they believe are their wrongdoings or actions to appease their ancestors [7]. These caregivers may experience guilt and shame, often neglecting their own needs and health. Others may feel overwhelmed by these beliefs to the point of failing to provide adequate care. Moreover, this view perpetuates stigma, which attributes blame and shame, thereby becoming a significant barrier to treatment [7, 13, 14].

Wilhelm Griesinger, a nineteenth-century German physician, was the first to declare mental illness as a brain illness [15]. He significantly impacted modern perceptions of mental illness and was a pioneer in community-based care for psychiatric patients at a time when most were confined to asylums in remote rural areas. Griesinger suggested integrating these patients into society and proposed that short-term treatment for acutely ill individuals could take place in city-based asylums connected to general hospitals. The significant advances in science, such as brain imaging over recent decades, have bolstered biological psychiatry and helped solidify the understanding of mental disorders as brain illnesses [16]. The predominantly biogenetic approach to understanding mental illness has become dominant, shaping the perspectives of mental health professionals and influencing public campaigns aimed at improving attitudes towards the mentally ill.

2.2 Courtesy stigma of mental illness: A double-edged sword

The stigma associated with mental illness acts as a double-edged sword, offering both challenges and unintended social consequences. While advancements in science have greatly enhanced the understanding of the causes of mental disorders, supernatural explanations continue to be invoked to account for abnormal behaviours [7]. Perspectives that attribute mental illness to demonic possession, divine punishment, or other misconceptions stemming from a lack of understanding contribute significantly to the stigma surrounding mental health. This stigma manifests as prejudicial attitudes and discrimination against individuals experiencing mental disorders and their families [7]. The stigma experienced by families of individuals diagnosed with mental illness is referred to as courtesy stigma, stigma by association, or family stigma [17]. Goffman [18] introduced the concept of courtesy stigma, which refers to the negative effects faced by those associated with individuals who carry a stigma. This is particularly relevant for family members of individuals with mental illness, who often suffer prejudice and discrimination due to their association. Family members and caregivers of those with mental health conditions often confront the challenges associated with this phenomenon, which can significantly impact their social interactions and emotional well-being [7, 13]. Therefore, courtesy stigma impacts not only the diagnosed individual but also their family, influencing how they are perceived and their experiences. This form of stigma may cause family members to feel ashamed of their relationship with someone facing mental health issues. Consequently, these caregivers and family members may be inclined to withdraw from social interactions to avoid potential judgment or stigma from others [7, 17].

Families dealing with courtesy or family stigma often experience both public and self-stigma, adversely affecting their quality of life. Public stigma, often known as social stigma, arises when society supports stereotypes regarding mental illness and discriminates against individuals based on these beliefs [19]. Self-stigma occurs when individuals who are targets of stigma internalize this prejudice, leading them to accept and reinforce society's negative stereotypes about themselves [20]. The phenomenon of courtesy stigma varies significantly among families situated in diverse contexts. This variation can be attributed to the distinct stereotypes that communities hold regarding mental illness, which are influenced by their specific sociocultural contexts [21]. Different communities enact varying degrees of stigma, affecting the experiences of families dealing with mental illness and contributing to the social dynamics surrounding these issues. Understanding these contextual differences is crucial for addressing the stigma and supporting affected families effectively.

3. Intersection of CRS and courtesy stigma

Stigma is a complex social construct that describes how people seen as having inferior qualities are treated negatively and unfairly [18]. Goffman pioneered the study of stigma in the 1960s, describing it as an attribute that profoundly discredits an individual, rendering them tainted and devalued [18]. Negative stereotypes, labels, and discrimination are not only directed at PMI but are often extended to their family members through their association with them [7, 22]. Some scholars have argued about the effects of power dynamics on marginalized communities. One key scholar, Crenshaw, introduced the concept of intersectionality in 1989 to examine how power and oppression affect individuals with multiple marginalized identities [23]. This framework elucidates how intersecting social identities shape distinct experiences of both discrimination and privilege. Examining these complexities provides a nuanced understanding of societal dynamics and systemic inequalities [23]. Therefore, understanding how CRS intersects with the courtesy stigma of mental illness is vital to ensure that caregivers' unique needs, experiences, and challenges are acknowledged, allowing for the creation of more effective support services.

Caregiving is a complex role that involves juggling multiple, often competing demands [14]. Research highlights the difficulties faced by caregivers of individuals with mental illness, including the challenge of maintaining control and meeting their loved ones' needs, while also coping with feelings of shame and distancing caused by the courtesy stigma associated with mental illness [7, 14]. Research shows that caring for PMI significantly affects the mental and physical health of family caregivers. It also influences their ability to handle caregiving stress, increasing their risk of developing health issues like depression and hypertension [14]. Having a family member with a mental illness often heightens the pressure on caregivers to manage various aspects of their loved one's life, including financial, personal, and household matters. This can significantly amplify the overall caregiving burden [14, 24]. Additionally, family caregivers offer patients emotional and physical support, but they also must deal with the physical and emotional toll of the patient's disruptive behaviours, which can disrupt daily routines and limit their ability to participate in normal social activities [25]. Caregivers tirelessly supervise their mentally ill loved ones, struggling to balance the demands of caregiving with their own daily lives, which involve juggling multiple responsibilities at once [24]. Consequently, there is growing concern about their ability to handle and cope with the mounting responsibilities and demands.

Adding to the complexity of caregiving for an individual with a challenging and occasionally more difficult condition to manage at home is the fact that CRS is further exacerbated by the courtesy stigma they frequently encounter. This can lead caregivers to feel guilty due to courtesy stigma related to mental illness, which is a significant concern. This stigma often results in a lack of supportive social networks for caregivers [7, 14].

To this end, the growing recognition of family caregivers' needs has led service providers and governments in many countries to invest in programs and support initiatives aimed at helping caregivers manage the stress associated with their responsibilities [26].

3.1 How stigma amplifies CRS

Many family caregivers of PMI suffer in silence because of courtesy stigma, often fearing that their relationships, job status, or reputation could be in jeopardy should they disclose that they have an association with someone diagnosed with a mental illness. This can exacerbate their caregiving role strain, causing them to be less likely to seek treatment, resources, or take action to seek support for their mental well-being.

4. Leininger's transcultural nursing theory in dealing with stigma and CRS

The stigma surrounding mental health is not a colossal entity but manifests differently across cultures, influenced by diverse societal values, beliefs, and norms [21]. Therefore, it is crucial to comprehend these cultural diversities in order to develop culturally sensitive and effective interventions. Leininger's theory of Culture Care Diversity and Universality is appropriate for culturally competent care because it includes social structures such as kinship, cultural history, politics, economics, religion, lifespan values, philosophy of living, and geo-environmental factors that influence cultural care [27]. This theory was developed in the early 1960s by Madeleine Leininger and is one of the few nursing theories explicitly related to culture care [27]. Family caregivers of PMI have the right to receive support and care that respects their lives and cultural values, which aligns with the guiding principle of Leininger's theory of transcultural nursing [27]. The goal of this theory is to promote and sustain the well-being and health of a population, which aligns well with incorporating this theory into culturally competent care and support for family caregivers of PMI to encourage coping and improve the quality of care [27]. Applying transcultural nursing theory enhances cultural competency, which can prevent illnesses and disabilities in caregivers of PMI. This is achieved by addressing caregiver burden and courtesy stigma through culturally competent nursing care, leading to more welcoming and knowledgeable support.

Leininger's Sunrise Model provides a visual framework that can aid nurses in applying critical thinking and their nursing practice to incorporate culture and social structure in providing non-stigmatizing and culturally competent care for families and caregivers of individuals with mental illness [28]. The theory consists of three core modes of culture: culture care preservation or maintenance, culture care accommodation, and culture care re-patterning and restructuring [27]. Healthcare providers who integrate the three modes of culturally competent care can deliver safe, therapeutic, and meaningful care to diverse cultures. Increasing healthcare providers' understanding of how the courtesy stigma of mental illness intersects with CRS can guide preventive and promotional efforts using Leininger's theory of transcultural care. Thus, enhancing healthcare providers' ability to understand how to address, meet health needs, and support caregivers of PMI fosters culturally congruent care that aligns with Leininger's theory.

When applying Leininger's Transcultural Nursing Theory to the care and support of families of caregivers for PMI, the focus can be on both emic and etic care knowledge. Leininger introduced emic care, which involves understanding culture from an insider's perspective, and etic care, which is an objective, external view [28]. Emic knowledge comes directly from cultural informants because they understand and practice support and care within the framework of their cultural beliefs and value systems [27]. On the contrary, etic care knowledge is derived from perspectives outside beliefs and values that are non-indigenous [27]. Thus, as posited by Leininger [27], healthcare providers can offer culturally competent care practices entrenched in emic and etic care values to maximize health and wellness, reduce culturally related stresses caused by role strain and courtesy stigma of mental illness, promote activities that ease role care burden, and improve quality of life. Furthermore, healthcare providers can gain more knowledge from available community resources, training, and through their experiences in supporting or caring for family caregivers of people living with mental illness, which is directly in line with the transcultural nursing theory.

5. Coping mechanisms for caregivers

The identification of effective coping strategies to lessen CRS in caring for PMI is indispensable. The significance of managing stress and the use of coping strategies cannot be overemphasized. Coping strategies consist of the behavioural and cognitive efforts to minimize, endure, or manage external or internal demands, as well as to ease the consequences of stress [29]. This encompasses the approaches and methods employed by individuals confronted with unpleasant or stressful circumstances, with the intention of either addressing those challenges effectively or ineffectively [30]. Literature indicates that family caregivers of PMIs usually grapple with engaging in appropriate coping strategies when faced with adverse situations [31]. Additionally, it has been discovered that family caregivers of PMIs tend to rely on ineffective coping strategies, exposing them to the risk of developing mental health problems and heightened stress levels.

The family caregivers of PMIs engage in both efficient and maladaptive coping strategies to deal with their challenges [32]. The diverse coping strategies are categorized into two classes: emotion-focused and problem-focused strategies [33]. Problem-focused coping entails practically addressing the stressor or problem by employing problem-solving skills to eliminate or weaken the stressor from the atmosphere. This involves coming up with solutions such as using effective communication skills to amend inauspicious circumstances, searching for information, considering the advantages and disadvantages, and taking decisive action [34]. Problem-focused coping strategies have been conventionally associated with improved mental and physical health, as well as reducing CRS, leading to enhanced patient coping [35].

Providing care to a person with mental illness can be emotionally and physically challenging, predisposing family caregivers to, among other issues, fatigue, muscle injuries, and exhaustion. Family caregivers engage in various approaches to mitigate CRS, one of which is engaging in exercise and physical activities, which have a positive bearing on the mental and physical well-being of family caregivers caring for PMI [36]. Moreover, family caregivers of PMI engage in counselling activities to achieve a decent and stable mental state to perform the caregiving role proficiently [14]. Additionally, they experience an ominous need for positive feelings relating to the recovery of their loved ones diagnosed with mental illness. The quest for professional counselling from qualified personnel is one of the central steps towards dealing with the strain of caring for a person diagnosed with mental illness [37]. Family caregivers who participate in stress management training tend to experience heightened levels of positive emotions [38].

Engaging in peer support groups is one of the critical essentials that aid family caregivers in coping with the strain of the caregiver role [39]. Peer support networks substantially enable family caregivers to share their challenges associated with caregiving and acquire knowledge about mental health issues [39]. Support groups are conducted in various arrangements and are intended to encourage social interaction for caregivers and those living with mental illness under their care, eventually improving their quality of life [14].

Family caregivers of PMI usually grapple with the demands of their caregiving role. To mitigate this, they need to access information to aid in bridging the knowledge gap on mental health. Precisely, they need information about the patient's diagnosis, prognosis, and how to manage their condition. Research indicates that understanding issues surrounding mental illness is closely associated with the quality of life for caregivers. Furthermore, insufficient knowledge can lead to heightened feelings of caregiving role strain, while a profound understanding can assist caregivers in appreciating their loved one's mental health issues and accepting the situation. Providing psychoeducation can assist caregivers by equipping them with information about the condition, psychological support, strategies for managing it, and techniques for coping with stress. This, in turn, can enhance their caregiving skills, strengthen their capacity to care, and lessen the burden of caregiving.

Although problem-focused activities' intention is to confront the matter head-on, emotion-focused coping is more about alleviating the caregiving burden that often comes with stress and comprises a broad range of strategies. People might isolate and distance themselves, shift blame, express themselves to others, meditate, or exercise. When confronted with circumstances that cannot be changed, individuals are more likely to engage in emotion-focused coping strategies rather than problem-focused coping strategies. Meanwhile, less effective emotion-focused strategies necessitate caregivers to manage their emotional response to stress through behaviours such as resignation or avoidance [34]. Several factors appear to influence caregivers' preferences for one coping strategy over another. In terms of emotional focus, individuals who interpret the situation differently without changing their actual circumstances, such as those who use resignation, coercion, or avoidance rather than changing their circumstances, are thought to struggle more and have a higher relapse rate when dealing with stressful situations [40].

6. Advocacy and awareness

Living with mental illness attracts stigma, which makes the experience worse than the condition itself [41]. The mental health stigma does not end with the patients diagnosed with the disorder but also extends to their caregivers. Stigma is an undesirable way of labelling individuals or a group of people excluded from society because of psychological, physical, or perceived differences [42]. This phenomenon places people living with mental illness and their caregivers in a stereotypical group, and the discrimination they experience hinders them from seeking clinical intervention [43]. The importance of tackling interventions to address mental illness stigma cannot be overemphasized because of the severity of its consequences, rather than simply reflecting on stigma manifestations and their effects. Over the past few years, as a way of actively alleviating stigma surrounding mental illness, the research focus has shifted to managing the stigma through intervention programs [44].

Extant literature emphasizes managing mental illness stigma through programs that involve people with lived experiences of the stigma, specifically the people living with mental illness and their caregivers [41]. The focus has shifted from programs representing mental health professionals, as they are seen as driving the mental health services agenda instead of prioritizing the welfare of the people with lived experiences [45]. Corrigan [46] argues that the effectiveness of programs addressing stigma related to mental illness depends on the collaboration between mental health professionals and people with lived experiences, as it allows unswerving or parasocial interactions between the affected individuals and the public. Shahwan [41] indicates that the views of PMI and their caregivers on addressing stigma can be broadly classified into four categories: advocacy, educational awareness campaigns, social contact, and legislative reform.

6.1 Advocacy

The mental health advocacy concept was established not only to promote the human rights of PMI but also to mitigate the stigma and discrimination attached to the illness [47]. Advocacy is crucial in that it serves as the voice for the voiceless, such as PMI, giving them a platform to strengthen public services, mobilize and activate communities, and hold government officials accountable [48]. Furthermore, it has been described by mental health experts as a strategy to facilitate the accomplishment of treatment goals within the patient's context. Advocacy encompasses numerous actions aimed at overcoming the primary structural and attitudinal barriers to achieving positive mental health outcomes in society [47]. Advocacy has been praised for its orientation towards both protecting negative rights and promoting positive rights [49].

6.2 Educational awareness campaigns

Awareness campaigns through public education can be an instrumental strategy in dismantling information distortions about mental disorders. It is an appealing approach to mitigating mental health stigma as it targets misconceptions and the lack of awareness, while at the same time fostering understanding of mental disorders through the provision of information [21]. [50, 41] suggested that young people are a target group for instructional interventions due to the increasing life pressures they encounter, the potential they possess to shape the future, and the opportunities that school environments offer for implementing interventions using a mastery approach. However, raising awareness among the general population can be conducted in various ways, although particular attention should be drawn to the likely problems that may emerge with media strategies due to their sensational presentation of stories [41].

6.3 Social contact

Public direct social contact with PMI and their family caregivers has the potential to significantly improve public attitudes towards mental disorders [51]. Many people in society have formed negative attitudes towards individuals with mental disorders because of the stereotypes surrounding these conditions, as they have never had close personal interactions with them [41]. Direct social contact can be facilitated through various approaches, including indirect, imagined, and direct contact. These methods are often employed to reach large numbers of people, as they are easy to disseminate and scale up, especially in massive campaigns [52].

6.4 Legislative reform

Legislative reforms aim to prevent all forms of discrimination, provide reasonable accommodations in areas such as education, employment, and housing, and enhance protections for individuals with mental illnesses [53]. Thus, safeguarding that PMI can enjoy the rights and freedoms granted by legislation and access remedies for unjust guidelines and policies.

6.5 Policy implications – supporting caregivers in a stigmatized context

Policy for caregivers of PMI is important, especially in the context of stigma, to address the courtesy stigma of mental illness, characterized by discrimination and feelings of guilt that heighten CRS. The policy can help in advocating for the necessary resources to support and empower caregivers. Policies can address systemic barriers that hinder effective support, helping caregivers avoid isolation, navigate complex systems, foster resilience, and reduce the burden of caregiving role strain.

7. Conclusion

The intersection of stigma and CRS is a complex feedback loop in which discrimination and societal prejudice against the mentally ill and their caregivers affect caregivers, leading to negative outcomes such as stress, over-caring to compensate for guilt, and isolation. Families dealing with courtesy or family stigma often experience both public and self-stigma, which adversely affects their quality of life. Public stigma, often called social stigma, arises when society supports stereotypes about mental illness and discriminates against individuals based on these beliefs [54]. Examining the complexities arising from the intersection of CRS and courtesy stigma can provide a nuanced understanding of societal dynamics and systemic inequalities, serving as a foundation for understanding the unique needs, experiences, and challenges of caregivers, thereby informing the development of better and more effective support services [23].

Author details

Keletwaetse Sakwape[1], Miriam M. Moagi[2*], Wada Gaolaolwe[1] and Gaotswake Patience Kovane[3]

1 University of Botswana, Botswana, Botswana

2 University of Limpopo, Limpopo, South Africa

3 North-West University, Potchefstroom, South Africa

*Address all correspondence to: miriam.moagi@ul.ac.za

References

[1] Gharavi Y, Stringer B, Hoogendoorn A, Boogaarts J, Van Raaij B, & Van Meijel B. Evaluation of an interaction-skills training for reducing the burden of family caregivers of patients with severe mental illness: A pre-posttest design. BMC psychiatry. 2018;**18**(1):84

[2] Sorayyanezhad A, Nikpeyma N, Nazari S, Sharifi F, Sarkhani N. The relationship of caregiver strain with resilience and hardiness in family caregivers of older adults with chronic disease: A cross-sectional study. BMC Nursing. 2022;**21**(1):184

[3] Liu Z, Heffernan C, Tan J. Caregiver burden: A concept analysis. International Journal of Nursing Sciences. 2020;**7**(4):438–445

[4] Cheng WL, Chang CC, Griffiths MD, Yen CF, Liu JH, Su JA, . . . Pakpour AH. Quality of life and care burden among family caregivers of people with severe mental illness: Mediating effects of self-esteem and psychological distress. BMC Psychiatry. 2022;**22**(1):672

[5] Cham CQ, Ibrahim N, Siau CS, Kalaman CR, Ho MC, Yahya AN, . . . Lee KW. Caregiver burden among caregivers of patients with mental illness: A systematic review and meta-analysis. Healthcare. 2022;**10**(12):2423

[6] Ebrahim OS, Al-Attar GS, Gabra RH, Osman DM. Stigma and burden of mental illness and their correlates among family caregivers of mentally ill patients. Journal of the Egyptian Public Health Association. 2020;**95**(1):31

[7] Gaolaolwe W, Manyedi E, and Serapelwane M. Family members' experiences of courtesy stigma associated with mental illness. Health SA Gesondheid. 2023;**28**(1):1–11

[8] Andersen MM, Varga S, Folker AP. On the definition of stigma. Journal of Evaluation in Clinical Practice. 2022;**28**(5):847–853

[9] Gurung D, Poudyal A, Wang YL, Neupane M, Bhattarai K, Wahid SS, . . . Kohrt B. Stigma against mental health disorders in Nepal conceptualised with a 'what matters most'framework: A scoping review. Epidemiology and Psychiatric Sciences. 2022;**31**:e11

[10] Müller T. Stigma, the moral career of a concept. Symbolic Interaction. 2020;**43**(1):3–20

[11] Clark E, Munday J, Watts A. Stigma, shame and family secrets as consequences of mental illness in previous generations: A micro-history approach. Health. 2024;**28**(1):74–89

[12] Ahonen M. Ancient philosophers on mental illness. History of Psychiatry. 2019;**30**(1):3–18

[13] Reupert A, Gladstone B, Helena Hine R, Yates S, McGaw V, Charles G, Drost L, Foster K. Stigma in relation to families living with parental mental illness: An integrative review. International Journal of Mental Health Nursing. 2021;**30**(1):6–26

[14] Sakwape K, Kovane GP, Chukwuere PC, Moagi MM, Machailo R. Exploring the needs of family caregivers of people living with mental illness: A qualitative study in Lobatse, Botswana. BMC Nursing. 2025;**24**(1):183

[15] Rössler W, Riecher-Rössler A, Meise U. Wilhelm Griesinger and the concept of community care in 19th-century Germany. Psychiatric Services. 1994;**45**(8):818–822

[16] Rashid B, Calhoun V. Towards a brain-based predictome of mental illness. Human Brain Mapping. 2020;**41**(12):3468–3535. DOI: 10.1002/hbm.25013

[17] Yin M, Li Z, Zhou C. Experience of stigma among family members of people with severe mental illness: A qualitative systematic review. International Journal of Mental Health Nursing. 2020;**29**(2):141–160

[18] Goffman E. Stigma. London: Penguin; 1963

[19] Thornicroft G, Sunkel C, Aliev AA, Baker S, Brohan E, El Chammay R, . . . Winkler P. The lancet commission on ending stigma and discrimination in mental health. The Lancet. 2022; **400**(10361):1438–1480

[20] DuPont-Reyes MJ, Villatoro AP, Tang L. Mechanisms of mental illness anti-stigma messaging matter: Leveraging mental health communication inequities among Latinx populations to understand what works and what we can do better. Social Science & Medicine. 2024;**349**:116865

[21] Ahad AA, Sanchez-Gonzalez M, and Junquera P. Understanding and addressing mental health stigma across cultures for improving psychiatric care: A narrative review. Cureus. 2023;**15**(5): p. e39549

[22] Stutterheim SE, Ratcliffe SE. Understanding and addressing stigma through qualitative research: Four reasons why we need qualitative studies. Stigma and Health. 2021;**6**(1):8

[23] Aaron SP, Waters A, Tolentino A, Rascon A, Phan C, Chen E, Travers J, Jones MG, Kent-Marvick J, Thomas Hebdon M. Complex identities, intersectionality and research approaches in millennial family caregivers in the United States. Journal of Advanced Nursing. 2023;**79**(5):1724–1734

[24] Alyafei AH, Alqunaibet T, Mansour H, Ali A, Billings J. The experiences of family caregivers of people with severe mental illness in the Middle East: A systematic review and meta-synthesis of qualitative data. Plos One. 2021;**16**(7):e0254351

[25] Addo R, Agyemang SA, Tozan Y, Nonvignon J. Economic burden of caregiving for persons with severe mental illness in sub-Saharan Africa: A systematic review. PloS One. 2018;**13**(8):e0199830

[26] Chen L, Zhao Y, Tang J, Jin G, Liu Y, Zhao X, Chen C, Lu X. The burden, support and needs of primary family caregivers of people experiencing schizophrenia in Beijing communities: A qualitative study. BMC Psychiatry. 2019;**19**(1):75

[27] Leininger M. Theoretical questions and concerns: Response from the theory of culture care diversity and universality perspective. Nursing Science Quarterly. 2007;**20**(1):9–13

[28] Limjuco Woodruff LA, Moceri JT, Tran DMT. Adapting leininger's sunrise model to understand the culture of clinical teaching. Journal of Transcultural Nursing. 2025. DOI: 10.1177/10436596251371692

[29] Folkman S, Lazarus RS, Gruen RJ, DeLongis A. Appraisal, coping, health status, and psychological symptoms.

Journal of Personality and Social Psychology. 1986;**50**(3):571

[30] Marzban A, Fereidooni-Moghadam M, Ghezelbash S. Coping strategies among family caregivers of patients with chronic mental disorders: A cross-sectional study. Jundishapur Journal of Chronic Disease Care. 2024;**13**(2):102–110

[31] Rahmani F, Ranjbar F, Hosseinzadeh M, Razavi SS, Dickens GL, Vahidi M. Coping strategies of family caregivers of patients with schizophrenia in Iran: A cross-sectional survey. International Journal of Nursing Sciences. 2019;**6**(2):148–153

[32] Bademli K, Lök N. Feelings, thoughts and experiences of caregivers of patients with schizophrenia. International Journal of Social Psychiatry. 2020;**66**(5):452–459

[33] Lazarus RS, Folkman S. Stress, Appraisal, and Coping. New York: Springer publishing company; 1984

[34] Mohamed RS, Mahmoud NZ, Mahmoud DAM, Eissa MF, Zohdy YW, Hafez YSR. Coping strategies and burden stress in caregivers of patients with schizophrenia and patients with bipolar disorder. Middle East Current Psychiatry. 2023;**30**(1):102

[35] Munroe M, Al-Refae M, Chan HW, Ferrari M. Using self-compassion to grow in the face of trauma: The role of positive reframing and problem-focused coping strategies. Psychological Trauma: Theory, Research, Practice, and Policy. 2022;**14**(S1):S157

[36] Cardoso C, Lumini MJ, Martins T. Effects of physical exercise in reducing caregivers burden: A systematic review. Frontiers in Public Health. 2025;**13**:1474913

[37] Olawande TI, Ajayi MP, Amoo EO, Iruonagbe CT. Variations in family attitudes towards coping with people living with mental illness. Open Access Macedonian Journal of Medical Sciences. 2019;**7**(12):2010

[38] Hajisadeghian R, Ghezelbash S, Mehrabi T. The effects of a psychosocial support program on perceived stress of family caregivers of patients with mental disorders. Iranian Journal of Nursing and Midwifery Research. 2021;**26**(1):47–53

[39] De Jesus NS, Maurice A. Exploring mental health carers' caregiving experiences in France. The Journal of Mental Health Training, Education and Practice. 2020;**15**(4):207–221

[40] Hedge A, Chakrabarti S, Grover S. Caregiver distress in schizophrenia and mood disorders: The role of illness-related stressors and caregiver-related factors. Nordic Journal of Psychiatry. 2019;**73**(1):64–72

[41] Shahwan S, Goh CMJ, Tan GTH, Ong WJ, Chong SA, Subramaniam M. Strategies to reduce mental illness stigma: Perspectives of people with lived experience and caregivers. International Journal of Environmental Research and Public Health. 2022;**19**(3):1632

[42] Okobi S, Bergeria CL, Huhn AS, Dunn KE. Evaluation of stigma related to perceived risk for coronavirus-19 transmission relative to the other stigmatized conditions opioid use and depression. Frontiers in Psychiatry. 2022;**13**:803998

[43] Hajizadeh A, Amini H, Heydari M, Rajabi F. How to combat stigma surrounding mental health disorders: A scoping review of the experiences of different stakeholders. BMC Psychiatry. 2024;**24**(1):782

[44] Morgan AJ, Reavley NJ, Ross A, San Too L, Jorm AF. Interventions to reduce stigma towards people with severe mental illness: Systematic review and meta-analysis. Journal of Psychiatric Research. 2018;**103**:120–133

[45] Ashton LJ, Gordon SE, Reeves RA. Key ingredients—target groups, methods and messages, and evaluation—of local-level, public interventions to counter stigma and discrimination: A lived experience informed selective narrative literature review. Community Mental Health Journal. 2018;**54**(3):312–333. DOI: 10.1007/s10597-017-0189-5

[46] Corrigan PW. Lessons learned from unintended consequences about erasing the stigma of mental illness. World Psychiatry. 2016;**15**(1):67–73

[47] Saha G. Advocacy in mental health. Indian Journal of Psychiatry. 2021;**63**(6):523–526

[48] Marshall-Lee ED, Hinger C, Popovic R, Miller Roberts TC, Prempeh L. Social justice advocacy in mental health services: Consumer, community, training, and policy perspectives. Psychological Services. 2020;**17**(S1):12

[49] Stomski N, Morrison P, Whitely M, Brennan P. Advocacy processes in mental health: A qualitative study. Qualitative Research in Psychology. 2017;**14**(2):200–215

[50] Chen SP, Sargent E, Stuart H. Effectiveness of school-based interventions on mental health stigmatization. In: Leschied AW, Saklofske DH, Flett GL, Eds. Handbook of School-based Mental Health Promotion: An Evidence-informed Framework for Implementation. Cham: Springer International Publishing; 2018. p. 201–212

[51] Jorm AF. Effect of contact-based interventions on stigma and discrimination: A critical examination of the evidence. Psychiatric Services. 2020;**71**(7):735–737. DOI: 10.7448/IAS.20.1.21395

[52] Damsté C, Gronholm PC, Groot TD, Gurung D, Makhmud A, Peters RM, Hartog K. Social contact as a strategy to reduce stigma in low-and middle-income countries: A systematic review and expert perspectives. PLOS Global Public Health. 2024;**4**(3):e0003053

[53] Da Silva AG, Baldaçara L, Cavalcante DA, Fasanella NA, Palha AP. The impact of mental illness stigma on psychiatric emergencies. Frontiers in Psychiatry. 2020;**11**:573

[54] Corrigan PW, Nieweglowski K. How does familiarity impact the stigma of mental illness? Clinical Psychology Review. 2019;**70**:40–50